Neutrophils in Infectious Diseases

Edited by

Fabienne Tacchini-Cottier

University of Lausanne, 1066, Epalinges

Switzerland

&

Ger van Zandbergen

Immunology, Paul-Ehrlich-Institut

Germany

Neutrophils in Infectious Diseases

Editors: Fabienne Tacchini-Cottier and Ger
van Zandbergen

eISBN: 978-1-60805-023-9

ISBN: 978-1-60805-382-7

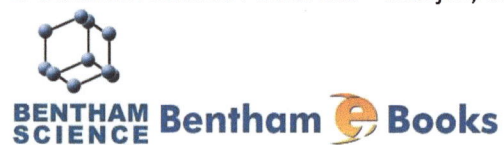

Bentham Science Publishers
Executive Suite Y - 2
PO Box 7917, Saif Zone
Sharjah, U.A.E.
subscriptions@benthamscience.org

Bentham Science Publishers
P.O. Box 446
Oak Park, IL 60301-0446
USA
subscriptions@benthamscience.org

Bentham Science Publishers
P.O. Box 294
1400 AG Bussum
THE NETHERLANDS
subscriptions@benthamscience.org

CONTENTS

FOREWORD

More than hundred years ago, Eli Metchnikoff was the first to discover phagocytosis by macrophages and "microphages", today known as neutrophilic granulocytes, as a critical host-defense mechanism. Their life-saving role in combating acute infections is undoubted as wittnessed by potentially lethal diseases resulting from defects in number or function of neutrophils, for example iatrogenic leukopenia or rare diseases like the leukocyte adhesion deficiency syndrome, chronic granulomatous disease or congenital neutropenia.

Historically, neutrophils were widely disrespected by researchers as gormless cells that crawl, eat and disgorge prepacked enzymes and reduced molecules of oxygen. This may have been due to difficulties in experimental approaches given the short half-life of the cells *in vitro* and *in vivo*.

Recent advances in technology have put the neutrophils in the centre of interest for infection biologists and immunologists. They are the first cells that are able to recognize tissue injury and the presence of genomes other than those encodes in the germline of the individual. Central to this function is to sense injury and "non-self" by pattern-recognition receptors, to send alarming signals to activate epithelial and endothelial cells, mast cells, macrophages and platelets. As key component of the inflammatory response, neutrophils are instrumental to recruitment, activation and programming of antigen-presenting cells by generating chemokines, regulatory cytokines and through direct cellular contact. In addition, they make important contributions to the activation of antigen-recognizing T- and B-lymphocytes and are thus important decision-makers and decision-shapers for the success or failure of the adaptive immune system in serving the collective good.

Some microbes like Chlamydia, Anaplasma or Leishmania are able to substantially prolong the usually short half-life of neutrophils (6-8 hours in the circulation, 15 hours in the petri-dish) by slowing-down the apoptotic program. Although the molecular basis of that interaction remains to be uncovered, it is clear that this mechanism paves the microorganisms to a silent entry into hosts cells and facilitates their dissemination through the organism.

Equipped with the "licence to kill" by means of the respiratory burst, the degranulation response and the formation of extracellular traps, it is not surprising that the killing machinery leaves collateral tissue damage in acute infections (pus), but also makes important contributions to the consolidation and the organisation of the extracellular matrix in the granulomatous tissue of chronic disease states with underlying infections, autoimmune reactions or tumors.

This e-book collects a fine selection of contributions from leading experts in the field of neutrophil biology in the context of infection. Their discoveries document that it is time to set aside the view that neutrophils are merely destructive cells that lash out blindly before dying. It is time to recognize neutrophils as life-saving body-guards which are in the centre of the network of the circuits that bring out the innate and adaptive immune system.

Prof. Dr. med. Werner Solbach

PREFACE

Host defense to intracellular pathogens depends upon both innate and adaptive cell-mediated immune responses. Polymorphonuclear neutrophil leukocytes which belong to the innate immune system are the first cells that are recruited massively within hours of microbial infection. Neutrophils are the main players in the killing of microorganisms and recently new methods of killing including nets formation have been described. Neutrophils mediate tissue damage at infected sites. By promoting tissue injury neutrophils contribute to the initiation of inflammation, which is now recognized as an essential step in launching immunity. The importance of neutrophils as decision shaper in the development of an immune response is only emerging as they have long been considered by immunologists as short lived, non-dividing cells, of poor interest. Now, neutrophils are emerging as key components of the inflammatory response, and are shown to have immunoregulatory roles in microbial infections. In addition, neutrophils were also reported to contribute to the recruitment and activation of antigen presenting cells. Thus early interactions between neutrophils and surrounding cells may influence the development/resolution of both inflammatory lesion and pathogen-specific immune response. The impact of neutrophils on cells present at the site of infection are only beginning to be studied and deserves more attention.

In this e-book the reader will find updated information about the role of neutrophils in the pathogenesis of 1) bacterial diseases including sepsis, mycobacteria and Chlamydia infections, and of 2) parasitic diseases including leishmaniasis and toxoplasmosis. The role of neutrophils in the protection against microorganisms has largely been underestimated and, until recently, their role was mostly thought to limited to a "kill and die" response. New neutrophil mode of killing, such as their release of extracellular traps to kill extracellular bacterial pathogens, together with several microbial strategies designed to escape NETs are presented in Chapter 1. We will emphasize standard and advanced light microscopy techniques that allowed major advances in the understanding of neutrophil biology, through the visualization of the interaction of selected pathogens with neutrophils in living animals (Chapter 2).

The aim of this e-book is to provide an overview of the recent advances made in the field of neutrophil biology. It will provide a basis for understanding future development that will occur in this area, and provide the reader with a short overview of some of the exciting new directions in which neutrophil research is moving.

Fabienne Tacchini-Cottier
Ger van Zandbergen

CONTRIBUTORS

José C. Alves-Filho

Associate Professor, Department of Pharmacology, School of Medicine of Ribeirão Preto, University of São Paulo, Ribeirão Preto, SP, Brazil

Edgar Badel

Engineer, Institut Pasteur, Unité de Génétique Mycobactérienne, 25 rue du Dr Roux, Paris, France

Elena Bank

PhD-Student, Institute for Medical Microbiology and Hygiene, University Clinic of Ulm, Albert Einstein Allee 11, D-89081, Ulm, Germany

Volker Brinkmann

Senior Researcher, Max Planck Institute for Infection Biology, Charitéplatz 1, D-10117, Berlin, Germany

Martina Behnen

Post-Doc Student, Institute of Medical Microbiology and Hygiene, University of Lübeck, Ratzeburger Allee 160, D-23562 Lübeck, Germany

Mélanie Charmoy

Post-Doc Student, WHO Immunology Research and Training Center, Department of Biochemistry, University of Lausanne, 1066, Epalinges, Switzerland

Fernando Q. Cunha

Professor, Department of Pharmacology, School of Medicine of Ribeirão Preto, University of São Paulo, Ribeirão Preto, SP, Brazil

Eric Y. Denkers

Professor, Department of Microbiology and Immunology, College of Veterinary Medicine, Cornell University, Ithaca, NY 14853-6401 USA

Friedrich Frischknecht

Senior Researcher, Parasitology, Department of Infectious Diseases, University of Heidelberg Medical School, Im Neuenheimer Feld 324, 69120 Heidelberg, Germany

Matthias Klinger

Senior Researcher, Institute of Anatomy, University of Lübeck, Ratzeburger Allee 160, D-23562, Lübeck, Germany

Claudia Kuss

PhD-Student, Parasitology, Department of Infectious Diseases, University of Heidelberg Medical School, Im Neuenheimer Feld 324, 69120 Heidelberg, Germany

Tamàs Laskay

Professor, Institute of Medical Microbiology and Hygiene, University of Lübeck, Ratzeburger Allee 160, D-23562 Lübeck, Germany

Cristiano X. Lima

Post-doctoral fellow, Immunopharmacology, Departments of Microbiology Instituto de Ciencias Biologicas, Universidade Federal de Minas Gerais, Brazil

iv

Angelo Martino

Post-doctoral fellow, National Institute for Infectious Diseases-IRCCS, Lazzaro Spallanzani, Rome, Italy

Markus Meissner

Senior Researcher, Wellcome Trust and University of Glasgow, Glasgow Biomedical Research Center, Office b-613, Glasgow G12 8QQ, United Kingdom

Geneviève Milon

Senior Researcher, Institut Pasteur, Département de Parasitologie et Mycologie, Unité d'Immunophysiologie et Parasitisme Intracellulaire, 25 rue du dr Roux, 75015, Paris France

Sylvia Münter

Post-doc Student, Parasitology, Department of Infectious Diseases, University of Heidelberg Medical School, Im Neuenheimer Feld 324, 69120 Heidelberg, Germany

Jan Rupp

Professor, Institute of Medical Microbiology and Hygiene, University of Lübeck, Ratzeburger Allee 160, D-23562 Lübeck, Germany

Werner Sollbach

Professor, Institute of Medical Microbiology and Hygiene, University of Lübeck, Ratzeburger Allee 160, D-23562 Lübeck, Germany

Mauro M. Teixeira

Professor, Biochemistry and Immunology, Instituto de Ciencias Biologicas, Universidade Federal de Minas Gerais, Brazil

Danielle G. Souza

Associate Professor, Immunopharmacology, Departments of Microbiology Instituto de Ciencias Biologicas, Universidade Federal de Minas Gerais, Brazil

Fabienne Tacchini-Cottier

Associate Professor, WHO Immunology Research and Training Center, Department of Biochemistry, University of Lausanne, 1066, Epalinges, Switzerland

Nathalie Winter

Senior Researcher, INRA, U1282, Infectiologie Animale & Santé Publique, 37380, Nouzilly, France

Ger van Zandbergen

Head of the Immunology Division, Paul-Ehrlich-Institut, Federal Institute for Vaccines and Biomedicines, Langen, Germany

CHAPTER 1

Neutrophils and Extracellular Traps in Microbial Infections

Volker Brinkmann*

Max Planck Institute for Infection Biology, Berlin, Germany

Abstract: Decades ago, neutrophil granulocytes have been recognized as professional phagocytes. In their granules they store a massive array of antimicrobial enzymes and peptides which they can release either to the outside or into the phagosome, where phagocytosed microorganisms are quickly killed. Some years ago a different antimicrobial function of neutrophils was discovered: once stimulated, neutrophils can undergo a cell death program that induces massive structural changes and finally leads to the formation of Neutrophil Extracellular Traps (NETs), which can bind and kill microorganisms outside the cell. In this review, the current knowledge about antimicrobial properties of NETs is summarized and microbial strategies to escape NETs are discussed.

INTRODUCTION

Neutrophil granulocytes are the first line of the innate immune defense against invading microorganisms. They can effectively control microbes and use diverse mechanisms of pathogen clearance. Upon sensing the intrusion of pathogens into host tissue, activated epithelium, mast cells and resident tissue macrophages release chemokines like interleukin-8, IFN-γ and C5a that attract neutrophils. After the expression of the surface adhesion molecules E- and P-selectin on the luminal surface of activated endothelium, neutrophils in the vessels start rolling along the endothelium until they finally attach due to the interaction of integrins and the intercellular adhesion molecule 1 (ICAM-1) on the endothelial surface. After diapedesis through the endothelial vessel wall, neutrophils migrate upward the chemokine gradient to the site of infection and combat intruding pathogens. Phagocytosed microbes get killed by peptides like cathelicidins and defensins as well as by aggressive proteases (Neutrophil Elastase, Cathepsin G, Proteinase 3) or by reactive oxygen species (ROS) generated during the oxidative burst.

But neutrophils can also kill pathogens extracellularly by NETs. In recent years it has been shown that this structure is effective against Gram positive and –negative bacteria as well as against fungi and parasites. Quantitative analysis of killing efficiency in vitro indicates that NETs and phagocytosis have similar bacteriocidal efficiency. Phagocytosis is quicker, but dependent on the living cell, while NETs prolong the antimicrobial properties of neutrophils beyond their life span.

EVENTS LEADING TO THE FORMATION OF NETS

Some minutes after stimulation of neutrophils in vitro with the protein kinase C activator phorbol myristate acetate (PMA), the cells lose their globular shape and attach firmly to the bottom of the culture dish, probably reflecting the attachment to the endothelium. Upon stimulation, the multimeric NADPH oxidase complex is assembled at the phagosomal membrane, and already 5 min after addition of PMA, formation of reactive oxygen species (ROS) can be measured, which peaks about 20 min after stimulation [1].

Many physiological stimuli that lead to NET formation have been reported. These include proinflammatory stimuli like IL-8 or hydrogenperoxide, direct exposure of neutrophils to bacteria like *Stapylococcus aureus* [1], *Streptococcus pyrogenes* [2], *Escherichia coli* [3], *Mycobacterium tuberculosis* [4], hyphae and yeast forms of *Candida albicans* [5] as well as protozoan parasites like *Leishmania amazonensis* [6]. NET formation can also be triggered by single pathogen components like LPS [7], M1 from *Streptococcus pyrogenes* [7] or lipophosphoglycans

*Address correspondence to Volker Brinkmann at: Max Planck Institute for Infection Biology, Berlin, Germany; Tel: ++493028460318; Fax: ++493028460301; E-mail: brinkmann@mpiib-berlin.mpg.de

from *Leishmania amazonensis* [6]. Rapid NET formation was induced by platelets activated via TLR-4 [9], a process that could promote the trapping of bacteria in blood vessels.

The components of the signaling cascade(s) that finally lead to the release of NETs are currently under investigation. One key component is certainly the NADPH oxidase complex since production of ROS is absolutely essential for induction of NET formation after PMA stimulation. When the NADPH oxidase is inhibited, e.g. by Diphenylene Iodonium, no NETs are formed. Neutrophils from patients with Chronic Granulomatous Disease (CGD) lack a functional NADPH oxidase and fail to produce NETs, but NET formation can be restored by addition of hydrogen peroxide exogenously [1]. The absence of NETs could at least partly explain the severe immunodeficiency of CGD patients who suffer from recurrent infections even under antibiotic therapy. After gene therapeutic restoration of NADPH oxidase activity in about 30% of neutrophils, a CGD patient could control a life-threatening lung aspergillosis probably due to the restoration of neutrophil capacity to make NETs [10]. Mice that lack a functional gp91, one of the NADPH oxidase components, are also unable to produce NETs [11].

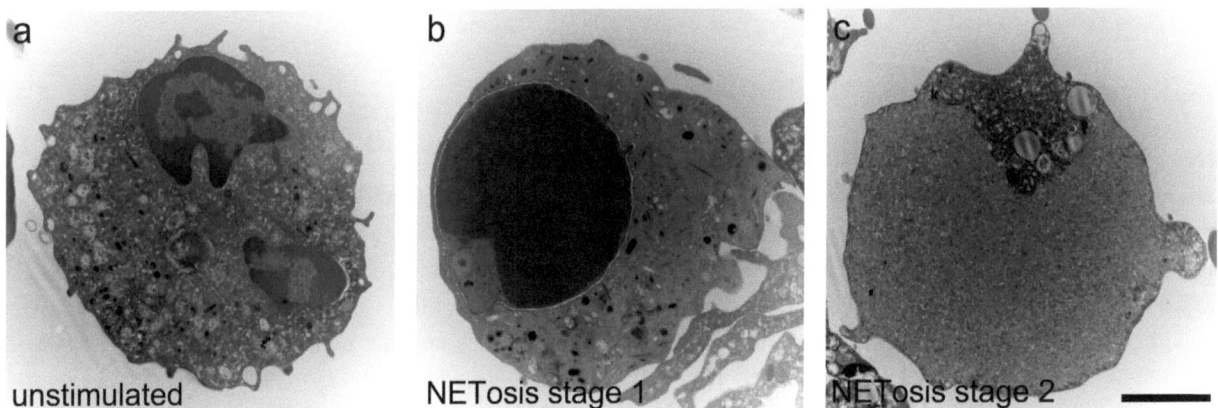

Figure 1: Unstimulated neutrophil (a) and neutrophils undergoing stages of NETosis (b, c). Bar = 2 μm.

Once the NADPH complex is activated, neutrophils undergo dramatic morphological changes. Nuclei lose their lobulation, decondense the chromatin structure and round up (Fig. **1b**) [1]. After about 2 h of stimulation with PMA, the nuclear envelope disintegrates into a chain of individual vesicles. Concurrently, granules gradually decay and finally the internal cellular compartmentalization is broken up. Thus, nucleoplasma, cytoplasma and granule contents are free to intermingle (Fig. **1c**) [1]. Finally, cells round up, contract and release their content when the cell membrane breaks. The process leading to NET formation is an active cell death program that is different from both necrosis and apoptosis [1] and has been termed NETosis [12].

During NET formation, relaxation and decondensation of the chromatin is indispensable and this is facilitated by posttranslational modifications like deimination of arginine to citrulline residues in histones. This process is catalyzed by peptidyl arginine deiminase (PAD4) which is stored in neutrophil granules [13]. Histone deimination in neutrophils is induced by proinflammatory stimuli such as LPS or hydrogen peroxide [14] – stimuli that also induce NET formation. In contrast, treatment of the neutrophilic cell line HL-60 with staurosporine or camptothecin to induce apoptosis did not lead to histone deimination [14] corroborating the observation that NETosis is a non-apoptotic cell death program. Citrullinated Histone 3 [14] and Histone 4 [15] have been identified as components of NETs.

During the final phase of NETosis, neutrophils appear to contract until the cell membrane ruptures at one point and the contents of the cell is expelled. It then spreads out around the remnants of the cell in a cloud-like fashion (live cell video accompanying [1]). NETs fill a volume that is several times larger than the neutrophil they were generated from and thus extend the antimicrobial potency of the living neutrophil both in time and space. It has been shown that Gram-positive, Gram-negative bacteria as well as fungi and parasites bind to NETs and get killed due to the high local concentration of antimicrobial enzymes and peptides [2, 6, 7, 16]. Binding to the NETs probably depends on charge. Incorporation of D-alanine residues to lipoteichoic acids of Streptococcus pneumoniae induces positive charge to the cell wall. Non-encapsulated strains without the ability to incorporate D-alanine residues to the cell wall are less positively charged and are more sensitive to killing by NETs [17]. Conversely, in a model system using rod-shaped gold nanoparticles with different surface chemistry, positively charged particles were more frequently found inside NETs [18].

EXTRACELLULAR TRAPS FROM CELLS OTHER THAN NEUTROPHILS

The formation of antimicrobial extracellular structures with a chromatin backbone is not restricted to neutrophil granulocytes from humans, various other mammals [7, 11, 19-21] and fish [22] or analogous cell types, e.g. chicken heterophils [23].

Mast cells after coculture with *Streptococcus pyogenes, Streptococcus aureus* or *Pseudomonas aeroginosa* or treatment with PMA release NET-like structures in a NADPH oxidase – dependent process very similar to NETosis. The structures contain DNA, histones and antimicrobial peptides (e.g. LL37) and enzymes (e.g. tryptase). In analogy to NETs, these structures were termed MCETs [24].

Work from one lab proposes a different mode of formation of extracellular DNA-containing structures both from eosinophils [25] and neutrophils [26]. Yousefi and coworkers propose that catapult-like release of intact mitochondria from living cells leads to deposition of extracellular DNA. After degranulation, granular proteins then bind to the DNA in the extracellular space. No mechanism that might permit the release of entire organelles from living cells is proposed, and it has not been shown if the extracellular structures contain histones – if the DNA were of mitochochondrial origin, it would not be complexed with histones and thus lack one of the main bacteriocidal components of NETs.

STRUCTURE AND MOLECULAR COMPOSITION OF NEUTROPHIL EXTRACELLULAR TRAPS

After their release, NET form huge three-dimensional networks consisting of smooth fibers with a diameter of about 15 – 17 nm which are studded with globular domains about 25 nm in size (Fig. **2**) [7]. Those smooth stretches probably consist of stacked nucleosomes, while the globular domains contain granular and some cytoplasmic proteins [27]. The backbone of NETs is DNA, and treatment with DNA degrading enzymes rapidly destroys NET structure and thus abolishes the bacteriocidal activity since only intact NETs provide a high local concentration of antimicrobial enzymes and peptides in the direct vicinity to bound microorganisms [7]. As will be discussed later, the ability to produce DNA-degrading enzymes confers greater virulence to bacteria.

During the last phases of NETosis, after break down of the nuclear envelope and decomposition of granules, chromatin comes into direct contact with most of the proteins expressed by mature neutrophils. Thus, it is surprising that only a very limited selection of those proteins and peptides are present in NETs. These include enzymes like neutrophil elastase, proteinase 3, myeloperoxidase as well as antimicrobial peptides (i.e. defensins, BPI, LL37). Extending the results of the initial description of NET composition which was based on immunofluorescence detection [7], a broader approach employing mass spectrometry on isolated washed NETs identified 24 proteins [27]. Interestingly, most of the cytoplasmic proteins were excluded from NETs with the exception of the heterodimer calprotectin, a member of the S100 protein family [27]. Although the bacteriocidal properties of histones has been known for half a century [28], only after the finding of NETs it became obvious how these nuclear proteins can interact with extracellular bacteria.

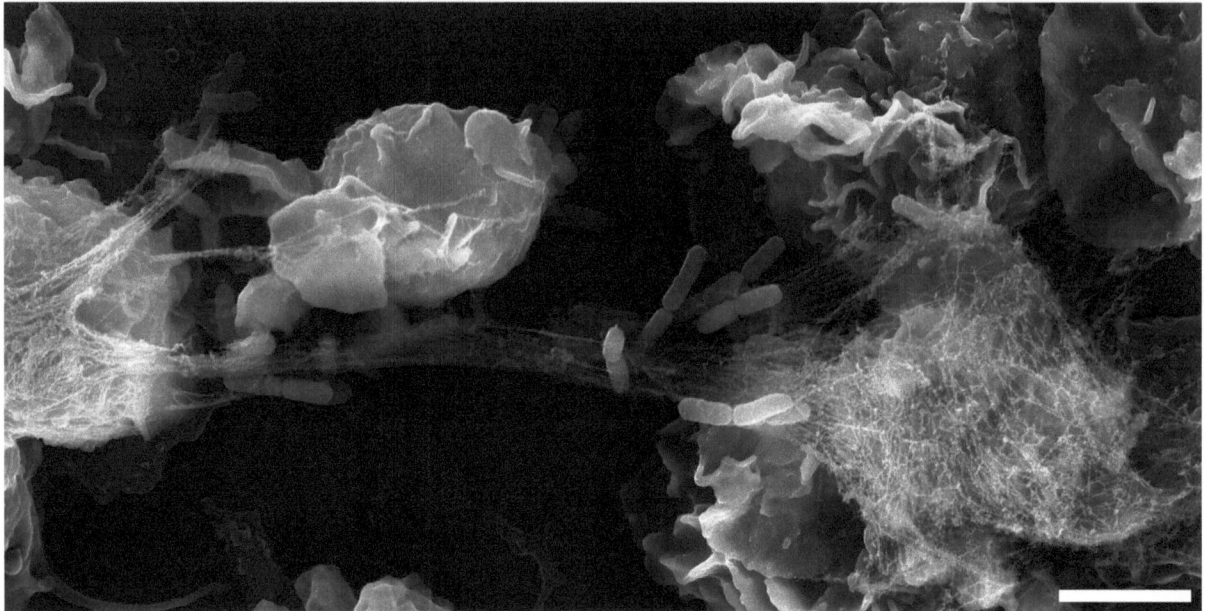

Figure 2: Neutrophil Extracellular Traps with trapped *Shigella* bacteria. Bar = 5 μm.

ROLE OF NETS *IN VIVO*

Bacterial Infections and Microbial Strategies to Avoid Neutrophil Extracellular Traps

Many pathogenic bacteria express extracellular DNases [29]. The benefit of this enzymatic activity and a possible role in pathogenicity has not been understood for decades. Sumby and collegues [30] were the first to provide evidence that group A *Streptococcus* (GAS) mutants that lack expression of extracellular DNases are less pathogenic than the wild-type parental strains and thus directly demonstrated that bacterial DNases are virulence factors. The GAS WT strain as early as 8 h after injection induced abscesses with necrotic neutrophils and obviously viable bacteria in the center. Numerous bacteria were present at later time points. In striking contrast, the mutant strain lacking all DNases was only present 8 h after infection. The lesions contained numerous viable neutrophils that cleared the bacterial inoculation. At later time points, no bacteria were detected. *In vitro* analysis of extracellular GAS killing by neutrophils revealed that the DNase-deficient strain was significantly more susceptible than the wild type strain. Although not proven directly, Sumby *et al.* proposed that the higher resistance of the DNase-expressing GAS strain is based on its ability to degrade NETs.

The direct linkage between NET degradation and bacterial pathogenicity was first demonstrated by Buchanan and collegues [2]. In a murine model of necrotizing fasciitis, they demonstrated that DNase Sda1 is both necessary and sufficient to promote virulence of Group A *Streptococcus*. After subcutaneous injection of wt M1 GAS, mice developed large lesions that contained about 100 fold more viable bacteria compared to animals injected with the Sda1-deficient strain. In purulent exudates from these animals, NETs could be demonstrated, while exudates from animals challenged with wt M1 GAS did not contain NETs. *In vitro*, wt M1 GAS was significantly more resistant to extracellular killing by neutrophils than the Sda1-deficient strain. In a gain-of-function experiment, Sda1 was expressed in *Lactobacillus lactis*. The resulting strains could effectively degrade NETs *in vitro*. After subcutaneous injection, Sda1 positive strains induced skin lesions more than double in size compared to control *L. lactis* strains. Thus, the expression of a DNase conferred virulence upon the otherwise inoffensive bacterium.

GAS has different means to prevent being killed by NETs. The most direct way to escape neutrophils is to counteract chemotactic attraction of the phagocytes. One of the chemokines regulating neutrophil migration is interleukin-8 (Il-8). GAS expresses the SpyCEP/ScpC protease that specifically cleaves Il-8 and thus prevents chemotactic migration of neutrophils to the site of infection [31]. The virulence of the mutant KO strain lacking SpyCEP/ScpC was clearly attenuated in murine infection models. If neutrophil recruitment cannot be avoided, GAS has means to inactivate the bacteriocidal cathelicidins in NETs by sequestering these small cationic peptides at the N-terminal part of the surface-anchored M1 protein. Thus, M1 protein induces NET formation, but it also confers resistance to NET killing [32].

Some bacterial pathogens, such as *Streptococcus pneumoniae* [33] are resistant to NET killing. Nonetheless, expression of an endonuclease (endA) promotes virulence. In a murine pneumonia model, WT pneumococci degrade NETs which allows them to spread from the upper airways to the lungs and from there to the blood stream. An isogenic endA knockout strain remains trapped in NETs and is far less potent in colonizing the lung. Thus, expression of endA allows pneumococci escape from NET confinement and to progress from a localized colonization of the upper airways to an invasive disease.

Pneumococci have alternative ways to counteract NET entrapment. Most pneumococcal strains isolated from the peripheral blood of patients with invasive pneumococcal disease have a thick polysaccharide capsule that protects them from professional phagocytes [34]. Non-encapsulated *Streptococcus pneumonia* strains were bound to NETs in significantly higher numbers than the corresponding encapsulated strains [17]. By inducing more positive charge to their cell walls by D-alanylation of lipoteichoic acids, Pneumococci gain higher resistance to NET killing by repelling binding of cathelicidins [17].

Mycobacteria like *M. tuberculosis* and *M. canettii* induce NETs readily and bind to NETs [4], probably due to their negative surface charge. Although *Mycobacteria*-induced NETs kill *Listeria monocytogenes* efficiently, even bound *Mycobacteria* are resistant to NET killing. Since in these experiments non-opsonized bacteria were used, the authors hypothesize that the signaling cascade leading to NET formation includes direct activation of TRL2/4 by mycobacterial cell wall components.

Haemophilus influenzae also survives contact to NETs. In a chinchilla model of otitis media, living *H. influenzae* bacteria were found dispersed in NETs, but encased by an electron-dense biofilm that prevents direct contact to noxious NET components [35].

Infections with Fungi and Parasites

Commensal and pathogenic fungi induce and are killed by NETs. *Candida albicans*, the predominant fungal pathogen especially in immunocompromised humans, has two propagation forms: it can grow as budding single yeast cells or as filamentous hyphae. Both forms are trapped in NETs and get killed by the granule contents [5]. Since *Candida* filaments are too large to be engulfed by neutrophils, NETs appear to be the only neutrophil killing mechanism against hyphae. While histones have been found to be bacteriocidal, they are not effective against eukaryotic fungi [5]. One of the main antifungal proteins in NETs is the heterodimer calprotectin [27]. This cytoplasmic protein lacks a signal peptide, and thus the export route was unclear until it could be shown that calprotectin is released as a NET component during NETosis. Calprotectin could prevent the degradation of NETs by microbial nucleases since it chelates the divalent cations which are essential for the enzymatic activity of DNases [36]. Indirect evidence for the indispensable antifungal activity of NETs was obtained after gene therapeutic treatment of a patient suffering from severe lung aspergillosis due to Chronic Granulomatous Disease (CGD) [10]. Patients with CGD lack a functional NADPH oxidase and cannot produce reactive oxygen species. Their neutrophils have limited antimicrobial potential both in phagocytosis and NET formation and thus CGD patients suffer from severe recurrent microbial infections. Gene therapy restored NADPH oxidase functionality in about 30% of a CGD patient's neutrophils and re-established NET formation and extracellular killing of *Aspergillus nidulans* conidia and hyphae. Six weeks after gene therapy, the patient had completely cleared the *Aspergillus* infection. Since hyphae are too big to be phagocytosed, the eradication of *Aspergillus* was most probably due to NET-mediated killing.

The presence of NETs in fungal lung infections has been demonstrated for *Candida albicans* [27] and *Aspergillus fumigatus* [37]. For both pathogens, NET formation is more potently induced by hyphae compared to other fungal growth forms. Interestingly, *Aspergillus fumigatus* conidia can suppress NET formation by covering the conidia surface with the hydrophobin RodA [37]. A different antifungal component of NETs is the soluble pattern recognition receptor Pentraxin 3 which is stored in specific granules and after NETosis is partly localized to NETs [38]. Pentraxin 3 – deficient mice succumb to infection with *Aspergillus fumigatus* [39].

The second group of nucleated pathogens which can be controlled by NETs are parasites. In a study with children undergoing a clinically uncomplicated Malaria infection, blood smears were analyzed for circulating NETs [40]. In specimens from all children, fibrous DNA-rich aggregates interpreted as NETs were found that contained erythrocytes infected with Plasmodium falciparum or free P. falciparum trophozoites. Due to the experimental set up, a direct killing of Plasmodium by NETs could not be demonstrated. An apicomplexan parasite of cows, Eimeria bovis, was found to directly induce and get trapped by NETs [16]. In this respect, viable sporozoites were more active compared to dead or homogenized parasites. The first direct proof that parasites not only induce but also get killed by NETs comes from a study with Leishmania amazonensis [6]. Leishmania and its surface lipophosphoglycan induced NET formation in a dose-dependent manner, and the parasites were killed upon contact to NETs.

CONCLUSIONS

In recent years, a multitude of studies have underlined the importance of NETs which have been found to be active not only against bacteria, but also against nucleated pathogens like fungi and parasites. During coevolution of metazoa and both prokaryotic and eukaryotic pathogens, bacteria, fungi and parasites have developed numerous ways to counteract NETs, from metabolizing signal molecules that would attract neutrophils to direct NET destruction by nucleases to employing shielding effects of capsules and hydrophobins. Although the impact of NETs during infection could not yet be directly studied due to the lack of adequate animal models, indirect evidence for the importance of NETs came from a CGD patient that after gene therapeutic restoration of NADPH oxidase activity could overcome a severe lung Aspergillosis. One aspect of NET formation, though, has not been addressed in this overview: If not tightly controlled, release of highly active neutrophil components can have severe pathological consequences. Thus, NETs are involved in a series of diseases ranging from infertility to autoimmune syndromes.

REFERENCES

[1]   Fuchs TA, Abed U, Goosmann C, *et al.* Novel cell death program leads to neutrophil extracellular traps. J Cell Biol 2007; 176(2):231-41.

[2]   Buchanan JT, Simpson AJ, Aziz RK, *et al.* DNase expression allows the pathogen group a streptococcus to escape killing in neutrophil extracellular traps. Curr Biol 2006; 16(4):396-400.

[3]   Grinberg N, Elazar S, Rosenshine I, Shpigel NY. Beta-hydroxybutyrate abrogates formation of bovine neutrophil extracellular traps and bactericidal activity against mammary pathogenic *Escherichia coli*. Infect Immun 2008; 76(6):2802-7.

[4]   Ramos-Kichik V, Mondragón-Flores R, Mondragón-Castelán M, *et al.* Neutrophil extracellular traps are induced by Mycobacterium tuberculosis. Tuberculosis 2009; 89(1):29-37.

[5]   Urban CF, Reichard U, Brinkmann V, Zychlinsky A. Neutrophil extracellular traps capture and kill Candida albicans and hyphal forms. Cell Microbiol 2006; 8(4):668-76.

[6]   Guimaraes-Costa AB, Nascimento MTC, Froment GS, *et al.* Leishmania amazonensis promastigotes induce and are killed by neutrophil extracellular traps. Proc Natl Acad Sci USA 2009; 106(16):6748-53.

[7]   Brinkmann V, Reichard U, Goosmann C, *et al.* Neutrophil extracellular traps kill bacteria. Science 2004; 303(5663):1532-5.

[8]   Oehmcke S, Mörgelin M, Herwald H. Activation of the human contact system on neutrophil extracellular traps. J Innate Immun 2009; 1:225-30.

[9]   Clark SR, Ma AC, Tavener SA, *et al.* Platelet TLR4 activates neutrophil extracellular traps to ensnare bacteria in septic blood. Nat Med 2007; 13(4):463-9.

[10]   Bianchi M, Hakkim A, Brinkmann V, *et al.* Restoration of NET formation by gene therapy in CGD controls aspergillosis. Blood 2009; 114(13):2619-22.

[11]   Ermert D, Urban CF, Laube B, Goosmann C, Zychlinsky A, Brinkmann V. Mouse Neutrophil Extracellular Traps in Microbial Infections. J Innate Immun 2009; 1(3):181-93.

[12]   Steinberg BE, Grinstein S. Unconventional roles of the NADPH oxidase: signaling, ion homeostasis, and cell death. Science's STKE: signal transduction knowledge environment. Sci STKE 2007; 2007(379):pe11.

[13]   Asaga H, Nakashima K, Senshu T, Ishigami A, Yamada M. Immunocytochemical localization of peptidylarginine deiminase in human eosinophils and neutrophils. J Leukoc Biol 2001; 70(1):46-51.

[14]   Neeli I, Dwivedi N, Khan S, Radic M. Regulation of Extracellular Chromatin Release from Neutrophils. J Innate Immun 2009; 1(3):194-201.

[15]   Wang Y, Li M, Stadler S, *et al.* Histone hypercitrullination mediates chromatin decondensation and neutrophil extracellular trap formation. J Cell Biol 2009; 184(2):205-13.

[16]   Behrendt JH, Ruiz A, Zahner H, Taubert A, Hermosilla C. Neutrophil extracellular trap formation as innate immune reactions against the apicomplexan parasite Eimeria bovis. Vet Immunol Immunopathol 2009; 133(1):1-8.

[17]   Wartha F, Beiter K, Albiger B, *et al.* Capsule and D-alanylated lipoteichoic acids protect Streptococcus pneumoniae against neutrophil extracellular traps. Cell Microbiol 2007; 9(5):1162-71.

[18]   Bartneck M, Keul HA, Zwadlo-Klarwasser G, Groll J. Phagocytosis Independent Extracellular Nanoparticle Clearance by Human Immune Cells. Nano Lett 2010; 10(1):59-63.

[19]   Alghamdi AS, Foster DN. Seminal DNase frees spermatozoa entangled in neutrophil extracellular traps. Biol Reprod 2005; 73(6):1174-81.

[20]   Lippolis JD, Reinhardt TA, Goff JP, Horst RL. Neutrophil extracellular trap formation by bovine neutrophils is not inhibited by milk. Vet Immunol Immunopathol 2006; 113(1-2):248-55.

[21]   Wardini AB, Guimaraes-Costa AB, Nascimento MTC, Nadaes NR, Danelli MGM, Mazur C, *et al.* Characterization of neutrophil extracellular traps in cats naturally infected with feline leukemia virus. J Gen Virol 2009; 91:259-64.

[22]   Palić D, Ostojić J, Andreasen CB, Roth JA. Fish cast NETs: Neutrophil extracellular traps are released from fish neutrophils. Dev Comp Immunol 2007; 31(8):805-16.

[23]   Chuammitri P, Ostojić J, Andreasen CB, Redmond SB, Lamont SJ, Palić D. Chicken heterophil extracellular traps (HETs): Novel defense mechanism of chicken heterophils. Vet Immunol Immunopathol 2009; 129(1-2):126-31.

[24]   Von Köckritz-Blickwede M, Goldmann O, Thulin P, *et al.* Phagocytosis-independent antimicrobial activity of mast cells by means of extracellular trap formation. Blood 2008; 111(6):3070-80.

[25]   Yousefi S, Gold JA, Andina N, *et al.* Catapult-like release of mitochondrial DNA by eosinophils contributes to antibacterial defense. Nat Med 2008; 14(9):949-53.

[26]   Yousefi S, Mihalache C, Kozlowski E, Schmid I, Simon HU. Viable neutrophils release mitochondrial DNA to form neutrophil extracellular traps. Cell Death Differ. [Article]. 2009; 16(11):1438-44.

[27]   Urban CF, Ermert D, Schmid M, *et al.* Neutrophil Extracellular Traps Contain Calprotectin, a Cytosolic Protein Complex Involved in Host Defense against *Candida albicans*. PLoS Pathog 2009; 5(10).

[28]   Hirsch JG. Bactericidal action of histone. J Exp Med 1958; 108(6):925-44.

[29]   Menzies RE. Comparison of coagulase, deoxyribonuclease (DNase), and heat stable nuclease tests for identification of Staphylococcus aureus. J Clin Pathol 1977; 30(7):606-8.

[30]   Sumby P, Barbian KD, Gardner DJ, *et al.* Extracellular deoxyribonuclease made by group A Streptococcus assists pathogenesis by enhancing evasion of the innate immune response. Proc Natl Acad Sci USA 2005; 102(5):1679-84.

[31]   Zinkernagel AS, Timmer AM, Pence MA, *et al.* The IL-8 Protease SpyCEP/ScpC of Group A Streptococcus Promotes Resistance to Neutrophil Killing. Cell Host Microbe 2008; 4(2):170-8.

[32]   Lauth X, Von Köckritz-Blickwede M, McNamara CW, *et al.* M1 protein allows group A streptococcal survival in phagocyte extracellular traps through cathelicidin inhibition. J Innate Immun 2009; 1:202-14.

[33]   Beiter K, Wartha F, Albiger B, Normark S, Zychlinsky A, Henriques-Normark B. An endonuclease allows *Streptococcus pneumoniae* to escape from neutrophil extracellular traps. Curr Biol 2006; 16(4):401-7.

[34]   Cross AS. The biological significance of bacterial encapsulation. Curr Top Microbiol Immunol 1990; 150:87-95.

[35]   Hong W, Juneau RA, Pang B, Swords WE. Survival of bacterial biofilms within neutrophil extracellular traps promotes nontypeable *Haemophilus influenzae* persistence in the chinchilla model for otitis media. J Innate Immun 2009; 1:215-24.

[36]   Corbin BD, Seeley EH, Raab A, *et al.* Metal chelation and inhibition of bacterial growth in tissue abscesses. Science 2008; 319(5865): 962-5.

[37]   Bruns S, Kniemeyer O, Hasenberg M, *et al.* Production of extracellular traps against aspergillus fumigatus *in vitro* and in Infected lung tissue is dependent on invading neutrophils and influenced by hydrophobin RodA. PLoS Pathog 2010; 6(4).

[38]   Jaillon S, Peri G, Delneste Y, *et al.* The humoral pattern recognition receptor PTX3 is stored in neutrophil granules and localizes in extracellular traps. J Exp Med 2007; 204(4):793-804.

[39]   Garlanda C, Hirsch E, Bozza S, *et al.* Non-redundant role of the long pentraxin PTX3 in anti-fungal innate immune response. Nature 2002; 420(6912):182-6.

[40]   Baker VS, Imade GE, Molta NB, *et al.* Cytokine-associated neutrophil extracellular traps and antinuclear antibodies in Plasmodium falciparum infected children under six years of age. Malar J 2008; 7:41.

CHAPTER 2

Imaging Neutrophil-Pathogen Interactions *in vivo*

Sylvia Münter[1,#], Claudia Kuss[1,#], Markus Meissner[1,2] and Friedrich Frischknecht[1,*]

[1]*Parasitology, Department of Infectious Diseases, University of Heidelberg Medical School, Heidelberg, Germany and* [2]*Wellcome Trust and University of Glasgow, Glasgow Biomedical Research Center, United Kingdom*

Abstract: This chapter gives examples of the use of standard and advanced light microscopy techniques to visualize the interaction of selected pathogens with neutrophils in living animals. To date the knowledge on the dynamic interaction of invading pathogens with immune cells is at the very beginning. We focus on recent studies of the parasites *Toxoplasma*, *Plasmodium* and *Leishmania* in laboratory mice and the bacterial agent *Pseudomonas* in zebrafish. In addition we discuss the basic imaging requirements and some technical pitfalls that can occur during image acquisition and data analysis. Advanced imaging approaches have become an essential tool in modern cell biology, which is also reflected by the rapid development of new high-tech equipment.

INTRODUCTION

Direct microscopic investigations *in vivo* arguably constitute the gold standard to probe the interactions of cells with pathogens. For example, a number of *in vivo* imaging approaches across the life cycle of the malaria parasite have not only confirmed *in vitro* data, but also helped to establish new paradigms that would not have been gained with the same precision unless directly investigated in a living animal [1, 2]. The design of an *in vivo* imaging experiment is complex as it implies freshly extracted organs or living animals. It necessitates prior knowledge gained by indirect biochemical and immuno-staining assays, which can give useful guidance for *in vivo* experimentation. Neutrophils constitute the major proportion of the white blood cells in the human body with almost 60% [3] and contain cytoplasmatic granules loaded with digestive enzymes. They are produced in the bone marrow and after final maturation they circulate in the blood stream. Unless neutrophils are recruited to an inflammation site, they circulate in the blood for up to 6 hours until destruction by induced cell death [4]. As a major component of the innate immune system, they build the first line of defence against invading pathogens [5]. *In vitro* it has been shown that it takes neutrophils about 15-45 minutes after sensing of tissue damage to fire off their arsenal of defence when they fail to encounter a pathogen within a short time [6]. This is about the time they need to leave the blood circulation and arrive at the extravascular tissue. At the site of inflammation or wounding they generate specific signals to retard their own accumulation and suppress their own activation to recruit macrophages [7]. More than 100 years ago Elie Metchnikoff formulated his theory of phagocytosis by observing cells moving inside transparent starfish larvae. He hypothesized, that protector cells inside an organism would mount an immune response against foreign matter. To test this, he mixed water fleas with spores of an infectious fungus and observed the engulfment of the spores into a membrane bound compartment. He could even further validate his theory in mammals (rabbits) that were exposed to anthrax [8]. At that time Metchnikoff was working at the Pasteur Institute in Paris. He started a collaboration with Jean Comandon, a pioneer of microcinematography, and in 1909/1910 the first ever surviving movie revealing phagocytosis of trypanosomes was made. Jean Comandon was probably among the first to capture dynamic images of phagocytosis and impressively showed the homing behaviour of neutrophils towards streptococci and bacilli [9]. In the 1950s one of the most striking films was made by David Rodgers, who captured the long chase of a bacterium by a neutrophil within a smear of red blood cells. This dramatic movie is featured prominently in the popular YouTube collection of science movies with an impressive 1,000,000+ views [10]. From that time on, live cell imaging in the field of immunology has become an essential tool for the understanding of the various functions of immune cells and their interactions with pathogens.

Upon infection, the ultimate goal of the immune system is the elimination of microorganisms. Two ways of killing by neutrophils are known: First they phagocytize by engulfing the pathogens and destroy them by phago-lysosome fusion. Secondly, once activated, they form extracellular fibres through the discharge of chromatin and granule proteins. These fibres accumulate and generate a network around the pathogen, hence the name neutrophil extracellular traps (NETs, [11],

*Address correspondence to Friedrich Frischknecht at: Parasitology, Department of Infectious Diseases, University of Heidelberg Medical School, Heidelberg, Germany; E-mail: freddy.frischknecht@med.uni-heidelberg.de

Fabienne Tacchini-Cottier and Ger van Zandbergen (Eds)

see also the chapter by Brinkmann). Interestingly, it appears that both killing strategies require reactive oxygen species (ROS, [12]), which are produced by NADPH oxidase. Net formation can be very abundant at the inflammation site and is necessary to distribute a high local concentration of antimicrobial agents around the infection site. By this mechanism a number of gram-positive bacteria e.g. *Staphylococcus aureus* [11] and *Streptococcus pneumoniae* [13, 14], gram-negative bacteria e.g. *Shigella flexneri* and *Samonella typhimurium* [11], fungi e.g. *Candida albicans* [15] and *Aspergillus fumigatus* [16] as well as protozoan parasites like *Leishmania amazonensis* [17] are trapped by NET formation.

Importantly, using live cell imaging it was possible to investigate the process of NET formation. It was shown that, once stimulated, the neutrophils become formless and eu- and heterochromatin homogenize. Later on, the nuclear envelop and the membranes from the granules collapse and enable the "clash" of the nuclear and granule components. The newly formed NETs are released when the cell membrane disintegrates [18]. This process, termed NETosis, is different from common apoptosis and necrosis as it is dependent on the ROS by NADPH oxidase [19]. Not unexpectedly, some bacteria are able to escape nets e.g. group A strepococcus bacteria (GAS) [20]. These gram-positive bacteria produce DNase and are able to degrade the chromatin rich NETs. Fluorescent live cell imaging demonstrated that GAS strains in which the DNases had been inactivated were more susceptible to neutrophil killing than the wild type strain [20].

MICROSCOPIC IMAGING

In order to study any part of the immune system it is advantageous to use non-invasive techniques without any tissue destruction. Live cell imaging now allows the conduction of *in vivo* experiments that require long imaging periods and can yield quantitative results. *In vivo* live cell imaging improved the knowledge on how immune cells interact with each other, their surrounding matrix and invading pathogens. For instance, it is possible to gain quantitative information about velocities from leukocytes in circulation e.g. neutrophils [21] and molecular distributions at the sub-cellular level [22].

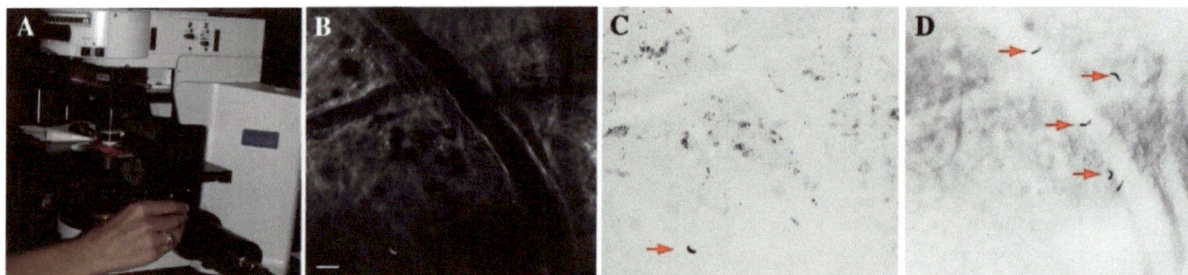

Figure 1: *In vivo* **imaging example.** (A) Image acquisition set-up to image pathogens or cells (in this case *Plasmodium* sporozoites) inside the skin of the tail of an anesthetized mouse under a "TriMScope", an upright two-photon (2P) microscope (courtesy of O. Selchow and LaVision BioTec GmbH, Bielefeld, Germany). (B) Collagen fibres visualized with second harmonic imaging inside the skin of the tail reveals blood vessels surrounded by collagen fibres. Scale bar: 20μm. (C and D) Two different planes showing naturally transmitted *Plasmodium* sporozoites (red arrowheads). Fluorescent cells of the host, e.g. neutrophils, could be observed in a different channel.

Today, pathogens can be filmed within tissues of living animals due to the advances in fluorescent labelling techniques, notably the expression of fluorescent proteins that allow detection of objects several hundreds of micrometers within a dense environment [23, 24]. Transgenic animals expressing fluorescently labelled cells have become available for a broad community. Especially for imaging neutrophils *in vivo,* a transgenic mouse line has been made that expresses an enhanced green fluorescent protein (EGFP) under the LysozymeM promotor. This label marks neutrophils, monocytes as well as macrophages, however neutrophils express higher levels of the reporter and can further easily be distinguished due to their morphology [25-29]. In combination with modern microscopes, this sets the stage for dissecting disease processes at the molecular and cellular level. Different microscopic set-ups range from simple widefield microscopes to fast confocal and light sheet-based microscopes. With the development of two-photon (2P) imaging, cell movement deep inside tissues (up to around 600 μm) is now possible, whereas standard confocal imaging only allows "surface" tissue penetration of about 50-200 μm [30]. Along with 2P imaging comes the possibility to visualize the surrounding tissue using second harmonic generation (SHG) imaging. SHG reveals only non-centrosymmetric structures (asymmetrical in three dimensions) such as collagen or muscle fibers (Fig. **1**).

2P imaging is based on the simultaneous absorption of two photons of twice the wavelength to avoid needless excitation. The illumination with light of a longer wavelength permits a deeper tissue penetration and further this light is less damaging to the surrounding tissue, thus inducing lower phototoxicity and bleaching of the fluorophore. However, comparing the energy deposited by 2P microscopy with the recently developed digital scanned laser light sheet-based microscopy (DSLM), it is still two orders of magnitude higher [31]. This can lead to cell death and has therefore to be carefully considered for any type of imaging since even an intermediate dose of energy can possibly alter the behaviour of cells *in vivo* (see below). A major drawback of 2P imaging other than high laser intensity and the cost of the system, is that the equipment is not easy to handle. It is therefore advantageous to use 2P microscopy in a specialized environment such as an imaging facility with professional maintenance [32, 33]. Therefore it should be carefully considered if such "heavy" equipment is necessary since bright signals e.g. inside the skin tissue can be easily imaged using fast confocal or even widefield microscopy.

NEUTROPHIL-PATHOGEN INTERACTION

In the following, we describe how four different pathogens have been observed interacting with neutrophils in different ways using diverse imaging set-ups and model tissues.

Leishmania – Neutrophils as Trojan Horses

Leishmaniasis is a disease transmitted by the bites of sandflies. Visceral leishmaniasis can lead to fever, liver and spleen swelling and anaemia, while cutaneous leishmaniasis causes skin irritations. A large number of species can cause the disease with *Leishmania major* being a main species causing cutaneous leishmaniasis in vertebrates. *Leishmania* parasites are transmitted in the metacyclic promastigote form and replicate within macrophages as amastigotes. For a long time it was assumed that macrophages take up metacyclic promastigotes after the bite, but it was recently proposed that neutrophils are their first host cells and that these cells can function as Trojan horses for the parasite transfer to macrophages [34, 35]. The parasites were shown to prolong neutrophil survival, and upon uptake of infected neutrophils by macrophages, to change their host cell. To directly probe these finding *in vivo*, a recent seminal study investigated the interaction between naturally transmitted fluorescent *Leishmania major* parasites with neutrophils and macrophages in living mice using a 2P microscopy set-up [28]. Direct imaging of *L. major* expressing the red fluorescent protein revealed that neutrophils accumulate in similar numbers at the site of a sandfly bite or syringe injection site whether parasites were present or not forming a plug that seemingly sealed the wound [28]. The study further confirmed that indeed neutrophils are the first to phagocytose *L. major* parasites despite an abundance of skin resident macrophages. Curiously, the movies showed many neutrophils passing by parasites rather frequently, pressing the question of how efficiently they recognize pathogens. Possibly the signal attracting them to the wound overrides whatever it is they recognize on the parasite surface. While moving rapidly to the site of tissue damage, neutrophils are about 20% slower after phagocytosis of parasites. This neutrophil slowdown is concurrent with the parasite uptake during migration. To probe what happens to parasites phagocytosed by neutrophils, one ideally would simply continue to image. However, one of the problems of imaging parasites after natural transmission is the large variability of parasite numbers, similar to what is observed during malaria transmission [36]. Further, fluorescent neutrophils continue to accumulate over time at the bite site and thus make it difficult to follow the parasite bearing neutrophils. In order to overcome this, parasites were injected by syringe into the skin of a mouse and infected neutrophils isolated and then reinjected into new (naïve) mice [28]. After this transfer, it was possible to visualize the release of viable parasites from apoptotic neutrophils close to surrounding macrophages. This infection-release-infection route was later termed the Trojan rabbit model [37]. In this model, the passage through neutrophils is of little advantage for the parasites prior to the uptake in macrophages in contrast to the Trojan horse model derived from indirect studies with human cells [37]. The large number of *Leishmania* species and subtle differences in their hosts might thus also indicate a limit of *in vivo* microscopy, as indeed human parasites might behave differently in human versus mouse tissue, and clearly the cells of the human and mouse immune system will probably do so, too. Nevertheless, this study highlights the tremendous power of *in vivo* imaging to study the role of neutrophils during transmission of an infectious disease agent.

Toxoplasma – Neutrophil Pioneers

Toxoplasmosis is a disease caused by the apicomplexan parasite *Toxoplasma gondii*, one of the most successful parasites that can infect literally all nucleated cells from warm-blooded animals. It is known that neutrophils interact with *T. gondii* parasites and provoke a protective effect by the production of interleukin 12 (IL-12) through the remodelling of the immune response [38]. In spite of this assumption, the exact function of neutrophils during *Toxoplasma* infection has not been elucidated. During an infection, neutrophils can migrate to the lymph nodes and possibly alter the immune response within the lymphatic system. Investigating the interaction of neutrophils with *T. gondii* using 2P microscopy directly within the draining lymph node [27] revealed the formation of highly dynamic neutrophil swarms in the subcapsular sinuses leading to a coordinated migration of neutrophils (Fig. **2**). Intriguingly, swarm formation was triggered by the egress of parasites fromed host cells and led to a clustering of neutrophils around the parasites. First so-called 'pioneer' neutrophils form small clusters and only minutes after the first formation, large-scale migration of cells into these clusters were encountered. This suggests that the small clusters only amplify the initial signal for cell migration. Following, the swarms are highly dynamic and two distinct types of swarms could be observed. Transient swarms contained only about 150 neutrophils and clustered together for about 20 minutes. In contrast to this, persistent swarms steadily grew over the imaging period and were finally at least double their size. Interestingly, the swarming neutrophils led to the removal of subcapsular macrophages probably due to release of tissue destructing metalloproteases. It will now be interesting to define the signals attracting and coordinating neutrophil migration and swarm formation and, ultimately, define their functional role during infection.

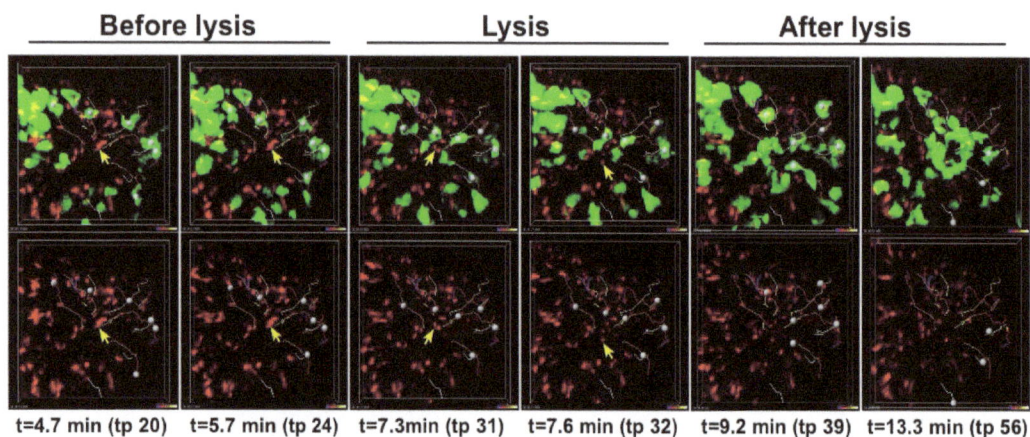

Figure 2: *Toxoplasma* **parasite egress co-occurs with neutrophil build up.** Neutrophils (green) and *T.gondii* (red) are visualized in a lymph node. The yellow arrows point to the position of intracellular parasites (before lysis) that burst from their host cell (lysis). This attracts more neutrophils. The tracks of neutrophils that enter the cluster are indicated as thin lines. Images were kindly provided by Tatjana Chtanova and Ellen Robey, see also reference [27].

Plasmodium – Racing in the Skin

Neutrophils and possibly other phagocytic cells were also shown to contribute to the destruction of another apicomplexan parasite and close relative of *Toxoplasma gondii*: the malaria parasite. Transmitted by the bite of *Anopheles* mosquitoes, the sporozoites of the rodent malaria parasites *Plasmodium berghei* or *Plasmodium yoelii* can be visualized during injection into the skin even by simple wide-field microscopy [1, 36, 39, 40]. Sporozoites move actively within the salivary gland to disperse in the narrow salivary ducts [39]. Once they are transmitted to the skin, sporozoites can migrate for several tens of minutes at speeds exceeding one micrometer per second on seemingly random trajectories through the dermis by using an actin and myosin dependent stick-slip motility [1, 41]. Quantitative analysis of the sporozoites' fate after transmission has revealed that they can invade both blood and lymph vessels and a large proportion of sporozoites remain within the skin, with some of them unable to move [36]. Even after 3 hours post transmission, individual sporozoites can still enter into the blood despite little movement within the dermis [42]. This appears to create ample possibility for phagocytic cells to detect and destroy sporozoites. Indeed, within the draining lymph node, where those sporozoites that entered the lymphatics accumulate, some have been seen in the vicinity of phagocytic cells, possibly dendritic cells, and indeed the parasites all vanish within a few hours [2, 36]. Visualizing *Plasmodium* sporozoites expressing the green fluorescent protein in the skin of living lys-GFP mice with a confocal spinning disc microscope revealed the interactions of phagocytic cells including neutrophils followed by phagocytosis of some of the non-motile parasites [43]. To date it is not known whether the data collected with the use of the rodent parasite model fatefully reflect what happens within the human host. As only very few sporozoites are transmitted during a natural mosquito bite, we would like to caution on conclusions, especially on possible effects of the presence of sporozoites on the immune system, gained from experiments where hundreds or thousands of sporozoites are introduced into the skin either by numerous bites or syringe injection.

Zebrafish as a Model Host

Model organisms to study cell motility *in vivo* include also transgenic zebrafish embryos. Their advantage over rodent models rests in their translucence, which facilitates imaging tremendously. Also, in the light of visualizing innate immune cells, it is of advantage that the adaptive immunity of the zebra-fish embryo is not yet fully developed [44, 45].

To investigate the mechanism of neutrophil-mediated inflammation, a transgenic line expressing fluorescent neutrophils under the control of the myeloperoxidase promoter (zMPO:GFP) was produced [44]. Vigorous tissue wounding induced an inflammatory response, characterized by the rapid directed influx of neutrophils at the damaged tissue. Time-lapse fluorescent imaging showed neutrophil motility in the transgenic embryo and proved that directed retrograde chemotaxis back to the vasculature is the regulatory mechanism resolving the inflammatory response *in vivo*.

Zebrafish embryos were also used in a study of systemic *Pseudomonas aeruginosa* infections in the neutropenic host [45]. *P. aeruginosa* is an opportunistic human pathogen that can potentially cause serious infection in those individuals with deficient or impaired phagocytes. Furthermore, *P. aeruginosa* cause ubiquitous chronic infection of patients with cystic fibrosis [46].

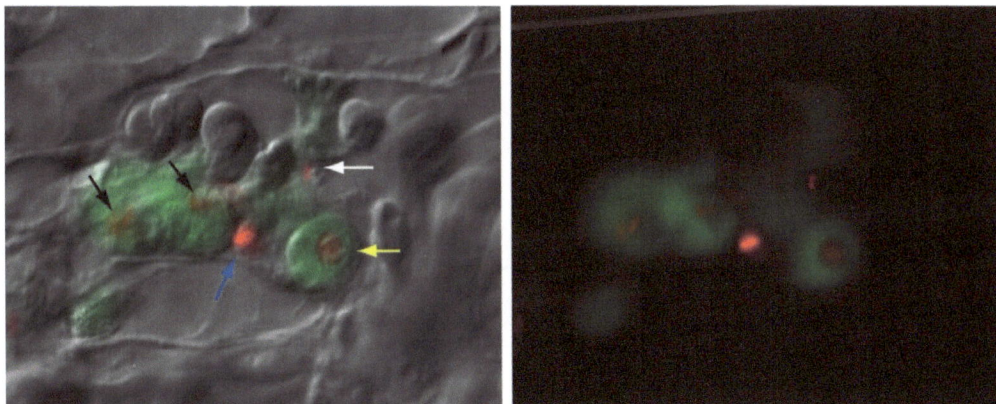

Figure 3: *Pseudomonas aeruginosa* **infection of a zebrafish embryo.** The myeloperoxidase promoter drives green fluorescent protein (GFP) expression in this transgenic zebrafish strain. GFP-expressing phagocytes are seen within the ventral tail of a zebrafish embryo infected with ~1000 CFU of mCherry-expressing *P. aeruginosa* (red), [shown with a differential interference contrast (DIC) overlay] at two hours post infection. Intact bacterial cells are seen within the vacuoles or adhered to the surface of two phagocytes (black arrow). A diffuse pool of red fluorescence, presumably mCherry released from killed bacteria, is seen within the vacuole of another phagocyte (yellow arrow). A bright red ovoid cluster (blue arrow) and an additional pair (white arrow) of bacterial cells that have not been endocytosed are also seen. Images were provided by Mark Brannon, J. Muse Davis, Jonathan Mathias, Anna Huttenlocher, Lalita Ramakrishnan, and Samuel Moskowitz, see also reference [45].

Based on previous work [44], differential interference contrast (DIC) and fluorescent microscopy was used to visualize *P. aeruginosa* infection in real time in transgenic zebrafish lines with fluorescent neurophils and macrophages [45] (Fig. **3**). This established that neutrophils and macrophages provide protection against a systemic *P. aeruginosa* infection. In order to identify the distinct phagocytes interacting with the red fluorescent bacteria, two green transgenic zebrafish lines were observed during neutrophil infection. After two hours post infection most of the bacteria are phagocytosed within neutrophils or macrophages. Moreover, red fluorescent protein (RFP) has been observed as diffused red fluorescence, signifying the start of the degradation process of the bacteria. Clearly, these studies on zebra-fish show that a carefully chosen, if seemingly obscure, model organism can be used to investigate defined host-pathogen interactions and yield valuable insights into disease processes. Similar to this, studies of innate immune responses in *Drosophila* gained tremendous insights into the molecules and signalling cascades involved in detecting pathogens, such as Toll-like receptors [47-49]. With the advent of whole embryo imaging [50] this could lead to a new wave of insights into host-pathogen interactions.

IMAGING PITFALLS

As the examples above illustrate, *in vivo* imaging is an essential tool to gain insights into the behaviour of pathogens and host cells in their natural environment. However, imaging without quantitative analysis and functional dissection of the observed processes remains at best descriptive, might overlook potentially important aspects of a given process or, at worst, might even lead to wrong interpretations.

It is therefore important to realize that all steps from image acquisition to analysis and interpretation of the data can be error prone.

For example, photo- and thermal damage induced by the illumination can be different depending on the microscopy set-up. Indeed, two orders of magnitude more energy is deposited within a specimen by 2P microscopy compared to confocal microscopy [31] and wide field imaging can be less damaging than spinning disc confocal microscopy (Spencer L. Shorte, personal communication).

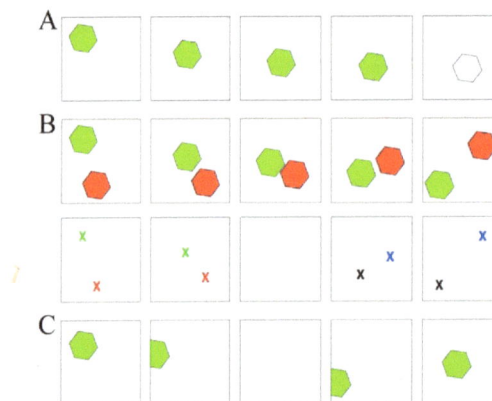

Figure 4: Challenges of cell tracking The cartoons highlight common difficulties encountered during tracking of motile cells. (A) Fluorophore bleaching leads to cell loss for tracking. (B) Fusion of touching cells makes it difficult to separate individual cells. (C) Movement outside the imaged region leads to the loss of information.

Therefore, if possible, one should test if the cells or molecules to be observed as well as their environment are robust enough to resist the stress induced by the illumination. The optimal microscope set-up has to be chosen accordingly and in addition, it is necessary to optimize the imaging parameters of each experiment to reduce the photo damage without loosing information. To this end, a recently established assay allowing the estimation of the impact of light on the multiplication of a *C. elegans* embryo is most welcome and should stimulate researchers to take these issues seriously (Spencer L. Shorte, personal communication).

Data analysis can also lead to artefacts and misinterpretation, e.g. if the individual signal is either weak or signals from two neighbouring cells cannot readily be separated. The latter case is illustrated for motile cells that need to be tracked (Fig. **4**). If they have the same fluorescent marker and are touching each other on their path, it is almost impossible for a standard computer program to reliably continue the track of each single cell.

Indeed, even for an experienced microscopist it might prove to be impossible to determine conclusively which cell follows which path. Similarly, the same cells can be attributed to two different tracks, when the cell is moving out of focus or the region of interest (ROI) and then re-entering it. In some cases it is possible to optimise the number of observed cells, *i.e.* imaging enough cells to obtain quantitative data but few enough to not impact negatively on the automated tracking result (cells do not touch or interfere with each other). However, when imaging natural environments this is not always possible and some customized tracking software might be required that takes into account information on the cellular trajectories or shapes to distinguish them and thus optimize the tracking results [51]. Alternatively, in some cases one can also try to circumvent these 'cell-based parameters' by using a step-based calculation. For example, within a population a few fast moving cells might move out of the imaged volume too quickly to obtain appropriately long tracks. In a step-based calculation the mean or median of all separate movement steps of the cell population in one experiment are analyzed independently to which track they belong [52]. This approach circumvents the 'cell-based parameters', where first all cells are tracked and the mean or median are given for the entire population of cells.

The above described challenges are limited to image analysis, but problems can naturally also arise prior to or during image acquisition (Fig. **5**). A very common problem occurring during the visualization of cells inside living tissue is a small drift of the specimen or the microscope stage. Thermal drift often accounts for a shifting of the microscope stage. This occurs due to temperature differences between the sample, e.g. a mouse heated with a thermal blanket, and the objective lens. It can be best prevented by building an incubator around the entire microscope, thus heating not just the animal to 37°C but the entire instrument too. A shift of the specimen during *in vivo* imaging of intact animal is frequently coupled to the breathing or heartbeat of the anesthetized animal or due to the perfusion of buffer over an excised site. If this drift is constant one can correct for it, for example by calculating out the drifts induced by heart beat [53]. In addition, signals from deep within a specimen can be distorted dramatically. These can probably be corrected in the future using adaptive optics [54].These are just the most obvious of technical challenges for *in vivo* imaging that should be kept in mind when adapting a new experiment to an imaging set-up. The best antidote naturally, is to talk openly to and enquire with colleagues and consult the wisdom of imaging facility managers.

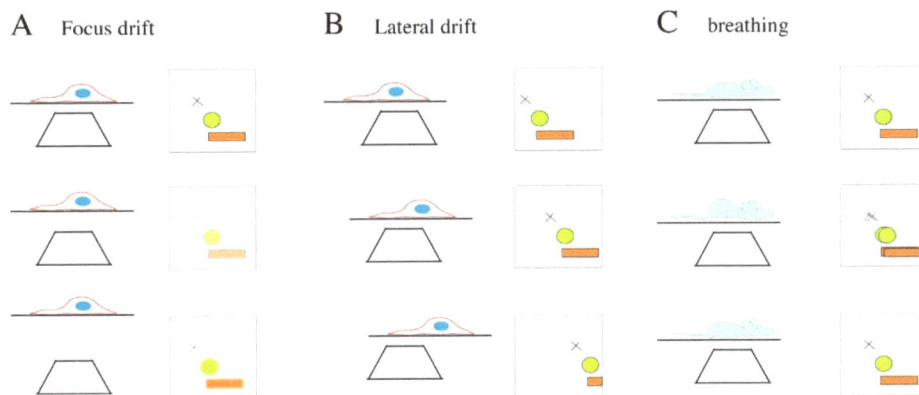

Figure 5: Challenges of *in vivo* imaging. The cartoon highlights some common image acquisition problems. A focus drift (A) most often occurs, when the microscope setup is not under stable temperature conditions. Depending on the magnification some little movement of the objective or the microscope slide, respectively, can lead to a blurred image. The lateral drift (B) is most often due to the mounting of the slide. As shown here, the region of interest is sliding out of the field of view. When performing imaging with living animal, one very often encounters problems with the breathing of the animal (C). Since the abdomen of the mouse is lifted and relaxed during image acquisition, the visualized object is also moving in z-direction. To circumvent this, one can either try to position the animal in order to avoid such strong movement or if the breathing is very regular the drift can be calculated out using heavy image analysis software.

ACKNOWLEDGEMENTS

We thank Ger van Zandbergen for motivation. Our laboratories are funded by grants from the German Federal Ministry of Education and Research (BMBF, Biofuture and NGFN), the German Research Foundation DFG (SFB 544), the EU FP7 Network of Excellence EVIMalaR, the Wellcome Trust and the Frontier Program of the University of Heidelberg. We gratefully acknowledge support from the Medical School and the Cluster of Excellence *CellNetworks* at the University of Heidelberg as well as the Chica and Heinz Schaller Foundation. [#]These authors contributed equally to this chapter.

REFERENCES

[1]　　Amino R, Menard R, Frischknecht F. *In vivo* imaging of malaria parasites-recent advances and future directions. Curr Opin Microbiol 2005; 8: 407-14.

[2]　　Amino R, Franke-Fayard B, Janse C, *et al*. In: Shorte S, Frischknecht F, Ed. Imaging Cellular and Molecular Biological Functions. Berlin-Heidelberg, Springer Verlag 2007; pp. 345-64.

[3]   Bainton DF, Ullyot JL, Farquhar MG. The development of neutrophilic polymorphonuclear leukocytes in human bone marrow. J Exp Med 1971; 134: 907-34.

[4]   Payne CM, Glasser L, Tischler ME, *et al.* Programmed cell death of the normal human neutrophil: an *in vitro* model of senescence. Microsc Res Tech 1994; 28: 327-44.

[5]   Kanthack AA, Hardy WB. The morphology and distribution of the wandering cells of mammalia. J Physiol 1894; 17: 81-119.

[6]   Nathan CF. Neutrophil activation on biological surfaces. Massive secretion of hydrogen peroxide in response to products of macrophages and lymphocytes. J Clin Invest 1987; 80: 1550-60.

[7]   Nathan C. Neutrophils and immunity: challenges and opportunities. Nat Rev Immunol 2006; 6: 173-82.

[8]   Metchnikoff E. L'immunite Dans Les Maladies Infectieuses. Masson and Cie, Paris 1901.

[9]   Landecker H. Microcinematography and the history of science and film. Isis 2006; 97: 121-32.

[10]   Frischknecht F. Infectious entertainment. Biotechnol J 2009; 4: 944-6.

[11]   Brinkmann V, Reichard U, Goosmann C, *et al.* Neutrophil extracellular traps kill bacteria. Science 2004; 303: 1532-5.

[12]   Hampton MB, Kettle AJ, Winterbourn CC. Inside the neutrophil phagosome: oxidants, myeloperoxidase, and bacterial killing. Blood 1998; 92: 3007-17.

[13]   Beiter K, Wartha F, Albiger B, *et al.* An endonuclease allows Streptococcus pneumoniae to escape from neutrophil extracellular traps. Curr Biol 2006; 16: 401-7.

[14]   Wartha F, Beiter K, Albiger B, *et al.* Capsule and D-alanylated lipoteichoic acids protect Streptococcus pneumoniae against neutrophil extracellular traps. Cell Microbiol 2007; 9: 1162-71.

[15]   Urban CF, Reichard U, Brinkmann V, Zychlinsky A. Neutrophil extracellular traps capture and kill Candida albicans yeast and hyphal forms. Cell Microbiol 2006; 8: 668-76.

[16]   Bruns S, Kniemeyer O, Hasenberg M, *et al.* Production of extracellular traps against Aspergillus fumigatus *in vitro* and in infected lung tissue is dependent on invading neutrophils and influenced by hydrophobin RodA. PLoS Pathog 2010; 64: e1000873.

[17]   Guimaraes-Costa AB, Nascimento MT, Froment GS, *et al.* Leishmania amazonensis promastigotes induce and are killed by neutrophil extracellular traps. Proc Natl Acad Sci USA 2009; 106: 6748-53.

[18]   Fuchs TA, Abed U, Goosmann C, *et al.* Novel cell death program leads to neutrophil extracellular traps. J Cell Biol 2007; 176: 231-41.

[19]   Steinberg BE, Grinstein S. Unconventional roles of the NADPH oxidase: signaling, ion homeostasis, and cell death. Sci STKE 2007; pe11.

[20]   Buchanan JT, Simpson AJ, Aziz RK, *et al.* DNase expression allows the pathogen group A Streptococcus to escape killing in neutrophil extracellular traps. Curr Biol 2006; 16: 396-400.

[21]   Zinselmeyer BH, Lynch JN, Zhang X, Aoshi T, Miller MJ. Video-rate two-photon imaging of mouse footpad - a promising model for studying leukocyte recruitment dynamics during inflammation. Inflamm Res 2008; 57: 93-6.

[22]   Nuzzi PA, Senetar MA, Huttenlocher A. Asymmetric localization of calpain 2 during neutrophil chemotaxis. Mol Biol Cell 2007; 18: 795-805.

[23]   Giepmans BN, Adams SR, Ellisman MH, Tsien RY. The fluorescent toolbox for assessing protein location and function. Science 2006; 312: 217-24.

[24]   Shaner NC, Steinbach PA, Tsien RY. A guide to choosing fluorescent proteins. Nat Methods 2005; 2: 905-9.

[25]   Egen JG, Rothfuchs AG, Feng CG, *et al.* Macrophage and T cell dynamics during the development and disintegration of mycobacterial granulomas. Immunity 2008; 28: 271-84.

[26]   Kim JV, Kang SS, Dustin ML, McGavern DB. Myelomonocytic cell recruitment causes fatal CNS vascular injury during acute viral meningitis. Nature 2009; 457: 191-5.

[27]   Chtanova T, Schaeffer M, Han SJ, *et al.* Dynamics of neutrophil migration in lymph nodes during infection. Immunity 2008; 29: 487-96.

[28]   Peters NC, Egen JG, Secundino N, *et al. In vivo* imaging reveals an essential role for neutrophils in leishmaniasis transmitted by sand flies. Science 2008; 321: 970-4.

[29]   Faust N, Varas F, Kelly LM, Heck S, Graf T. Insertion of enhanced green fluorescent protein into the lysozyme gene creates mice with green fluorescent granulocytes and macrophages. Blood 2000; 96: 719-26.

[30]   Helmchen F, Denk W. Deep tissue two-photon microscopy. Nat Methods 2005; 2: 932-40.

[31]   Keller PJ, Schmidt AD, Wittbrodt J, Stelzer EH. Reconstruction of zebrafish early embryonic development by scanned light sheet microscopy. Science 2008; 322: 1065-9.

[32]   Anderson KI, Sanderson J, Peychl J. In: Shorte SL, Frischknecht F, Ed. Imaging Cellular and Molecular Biological Functions. Heidelberg, Springer Verlag 2007; pp. 93-113.

[33]   Engel U. Imaging centers as partnerships between industry and academia: NICs go global. Biotechnol J 2009; 4: 797-803.

[34]   Laskay T, van Zandbergen G, Solbach W. Neutrophil granulocytes-trojan horses for leishmania major and other intracellular microbes? Trends Microbiol 2003; 11: 210-4.

[35]   van Zandbergen G, Klinger M, Mueller A, *et al.* Cutting edge: neutrophil granulocyte serves as a vector for leishmania entry into macrophages. J Immunol 2004; 173: 6521-5.

[36]   Amino R, Thiberge S, Martin B, *et al.* Quantitative imaging of plasmodium transmission from mosquito to mammal. Nat Med 2006; 12: 220-4.

[37]   Ritter U, Frischknecht F, van Zandbergen G. Are neutrophils important host cells for Leishmania parasites? Trends Parasitol 2009; 25: 505-10.

[38]   Bennouna S, Bliss SK, Curiel TJ, Denkers EY. Cross-talk in the innate immune system: neutrophils instruct recruitment and activation of dendritic cells during microbial infection. J Immunol 2003; 171: 6052-8.

[39]   Frischknecht F, Baldacci P, Martin B, *et al.* Imaging movement of malaria parasites during transmission by anopheles mosquitoes. Cell Microbiol 2004; 6: 687-94.

[40]   Vanderberg JP, Frevert U. Intravital microscopy demonstrating antibody-mediated immobilisation of plasmodium berghei sporozoites injected into skin by mosquitoes. Int J Parasitol 2004; 34: 991-6.

[41]   Munter S, Sabass B, Selhuber-Unkel C, *et al.* Plasmodium sporozoite motility is modulated by the turnover of discrete adhesion sites. Cell Host Microbe 2009; 6: 551-62.

[42]   Yamauchi LM, Coppi A, Snounou G, Sinnis P. Plasmodium sporozoites trickle out of the injection site. Cell Microbiol 2007; 9: 1215-22.

[43]   Amino R, Giovannini D, Thiberge S, *et al.* Host cell traversal is important for progression of the malaria parasite through the dermis to the liver. Cell Host Microbe 2008; 3: 88-96.

[44]   Mathias JR, Perrin BJ, Liu TX, *et al.* Resolution of inflammation by retrograde chemotaxis of neutrophils in transgenic zebrafish. J Leukoc Biol 2006; 80: 1281-8.

[45]   Brannon MK, Davis JM, Mathias JR, *et al.* Pseudomonas aeruginosa type III secretion system interacts with phagocytes to modulate systemic infection of zebrafish embryos. Cell Microbiol 2009; 5: 755-68.

[46]   Sadikot RT, Blackwell TS, Christman JW, Prince AS. Pathogen-host interactions in pseudomonas aeruginosa pneumonia. Am J Respir Crit Care Med 2005; 171: 1209-23.

[47]   Anderson KV, Bokla L, Nusslein-Volhard C. Establishment of dorsal-ventral polarity in the drosophila embryo: the induction of polarity by the toll gene product. Cell 1985; 42: 791-8.

[48]   Anderson KV, Jurgens G, Nusslein-Volhard C. Establishment of dorsal-ventral polarity in the drosophila embryo: genetic studies on the role of the toll gene product. Cell 1985; 42: 779-89.

[49]   Lemaitre B, Nicolas E, Michaut L, Reichhart JM, Hoffmann JA. The dorsoventral regulatory gene cassette spatzle/Toll/cactus controls the potent antifungal response in drosophila adults. Cell 1996; 86: 973-83.

[50]   Keller PJ, Schmidt AD, Santella A, *et al.* Fast, high-contrast imaging of animal development with scanned light sheet-based structured-illumination microscopy. Nat Methods 2010; 7: 637-42.

[51]   Chenouard N, Dufour A, Olivo-Marin JC. Tracking algorithms chase down pathogens. Biotechnol J 2009; 4: 838-45.

[52]   Beltman JB, Maree AF, de Boer RJ. Analysing immune cell migration. Nat Rev Immunol 2009; 9: 789-98.

[53]   Forouhar AS, Liebling M, Hickerson A, *et al.* The embryonic vertebrate heart tube is a dynamic suction pump. Science 2006; 312: 751-3.

[54]   Ji N, Milkie DE, Betzig E. Adaptive optics via pupil segmentation for high-resolution imaging in biological tissues. Nat Methods 2010; 7: 141-7.

CHAPTER 3

Neutrophils in the Context of Polymicrobial Sepsis

Danielle G. Souza[1,2], José C. Alves-Filho[3], Fernando Q. Cunha[3], Cristiano X. Lima[1] and Mauro M. Teixeira[1,4,*]

[1]*Immunopharmacology*, [2]*Departments of Microbiology and* [4]*Biochemistry and Immunology, Instituto de Ciencias Biologicas, Universidade Federal de Minas Gerais, Belo Horizonte, MG, Brazil and* [3]*Department of Pharmacology, School of Medicine of Ribeirão Preto, University of São Paulo, Ribeirão Preto, SP, Brazil*

Abstract: Sepsis is defined as systemic inflammation in the setting of infection. Sepsis may evolve to severe sepsis and septic shock, which are the end result of complex interactions between infecting organisms and several elements of the host response. The severe forms of sepsis are associated with evidence of organ dysfunction and high lethality rates. This chapter focuses on the putative role of neutrophils in the pathogenesis of sepsis. Neutrophils play essential roles in host defence through their ability to clear bacterial and other infections. To this end, neutrophils have to migrate to the site (focus) of infection where they will phagocytise and kill bacteria and release mediators, necessary for the activation of other cell types. However, failure of neutrophils to migrate into the site of infection may facilitate systemic dissemination of the pathogen leading to release of pathogen, pathogen-associated products and inflammatory mediators in the circulation. The latter, when in high concentrations in the circulation, can activate neutrophils and other leukocytes in the systemic compartment leading to damage of healthy tissues and death. In this chapter, we discuss some of the mechanisms which lead to dysregulated recruitment of neutrophils to the infection focus and their relevance to the development of multi-organ injury and severe sepsis.

INITIAL REMARKS

Sepsis was defined by a consensus statement in 1992 as systemic inflammation in the setting of infection. Severe sepsis is defined as sepsis plus sepsis-induced organ dysfunction or tissue hypoperfusion. If sepsis-induced hypotension persists despite adequate fluid resuscitation, septic shock occurs [1]. Severe sepsis and septic shock are the end result of complex interactions between infecting organisms and several elements of the host response [2,3]. The severe forms of sepsis are associated with evidence of organ dysfunction - ie, tissue hypoperfusion and hypoxia, lactic acidosis, oliguria, or altered cerebral function [2,3]. Indeed, multi-organ failure is the final consequence of severe sepsis, whatever the causative agent [4]. Despite prompt treatment with antibiotics, provision of adequate fluid resuscitation, and technological support of organ function, the world-wide mortality rate of sepsis is approximately 35% and has not changed significantly for over many years [5].

In sepsis, several factors are implicated in the pathogenesis of multi-organ failure, including the endocrine [6,7] and immune systems [8], disseminated intravascular coagulation [9], genetic susceptibility [10,11] and derangement of energy metabolism, possibly in mitochondria [12,13]. Several lines of evidence argue that systemic inflammation secondary to systemic levels of bacterial components or inflammatory mediators is a major cause of organ failure. Indeed, the septic syndrome is characterized by activation of several types of cells, including lymphocytes [14], macrophage [15], dendritic cells [16], endothelial cells [17], platelets [18] and neutrophils [19-21]. This chapter focuses on the putative role of neutrophils in the pathogenesis of sepsis.

Why are neutrophils relevant in the context of sepsis? Neutrophils play essential roles in host defence through their ability to clear bacterial and other infections. As mentioned above, bacterial infections are the most frequent cause of sepsis, and therefore adequate neutrophil mobilization and activation in tissue is necessary to deal with an acute infection. To this end, neutrophils have to migrate to the site (focus) of infection where they will phagocytise and kill bacteria and release mediators, necessary for the activation of other cell types [22]. However, failure of neutrophils to migrate into the site of infection may facilitate systemic dissemination of the pathogen leading to release of bacteria, bacterial products and inflammatory mediators in the circulation [21]. The latter, when in high concentrations in the circulation, can activate neutrophils and other leukocytes in the systemic compartment leading to damage of healthy tissues [4].

Address correspondence to Mauro M. Teixeira at: Immunopharmacology, Department of Biochemistry and Immunology, Instituto de Ciencias Biologicas, Universidade Federal de Minas Gerais, Belo Horizonte, MG, Brazil; E-mail: mmtex@icb.ufmg.br

Indeed, sepsis is characterized by accumulation of neutrophils in vital organs, including lungs [23], liver [24,25], kidney [26,27] and heart [8,28]. In these organs, systemic activation of neutrophils does not lead to their migration into the tissues [29,30]. Systemically activated neutrophils are trapped within the microcirculation where they can secrete free radicals, release enzymes and other mediators that may cause plasma extravasation, endothelial hyperactivity, fibrin deposition and vascular occlusion, which prevents oxygenation and leads to tissue damage [4]. Therefore, it is necessary that neutrophils reach the focus of infection and deal with bacteria. However, the highly destructive capacity of these cells also raises the potential for neutrophils to damage healthy tissues when they are activated in the circulation. Here, we try to understand some of the mechanisms which lead to deregulated recruitment of neutrophils to the infection focus and that facilitate the development of multi-organ injury and sepsis. We will initially discuss the current paradigm for neutrophil migration in acute inflammation. The relevance of deregulated neutrophil recruitment and why this phenomenon may occur in the context of sepsis will be discussed.

NEUTROPHIL RECRUITMENT DURING BACTERIAL INFECTION

The number of neutrophils in the peripheral blood is usually fairly constant, but the host is capable of markedly increasing numbers of circulating neutrophils. Indeed, there is a considerable reserve pool of mature neutrophils within the bone marrow which can be rapidly mobilized during inflammatory reactions, such as in the early phase of sepsis. Egress of neutrophils from the bone marrow results in a dramatic rise in circulating neutrophil numbers, which thereby increases the number of neutrophils available for recruitment into sites of inflammation [31].

The migration of neutrophils from the intravascular to the extravascular compartment predominantly occurs in the postcapillary venules and is mediated by a combination of mechanical, chemical and molecular processes (Fig. **1**). These are distinct events that are linked in a temporal sequence [32]. The initial step is "margination" or movement of the neutrophils from the central stream to the periphery of a vessel [33]. This process requires cellular interaction involving the surfaces of the neutrophil and endothelial cells, resulting in neutrophil rolling along the luminal surface of postcapillary venules. **Tethering and rolling** are dependent on both physical and molecular forces and are mediated by selectins and their ligands [34]. Selectins are a family of glycoprotein surface adhesion molecules, and include E-selectin (CD62E; expressed on endothelial cells), L-selectin (CD62L; expressed exclusively on leukocytes) and P-selectin (CD62P; expressed on platelets and endothelial cells). On the neutrophil surface, L-selectin interacts with specific oligaccharide moieties on endothelial-cell surface glycoproteins, whereas on the endothelium, E-selectin and P-selectin similarly recognize specific neutrophil carbohydrate motifs [34].

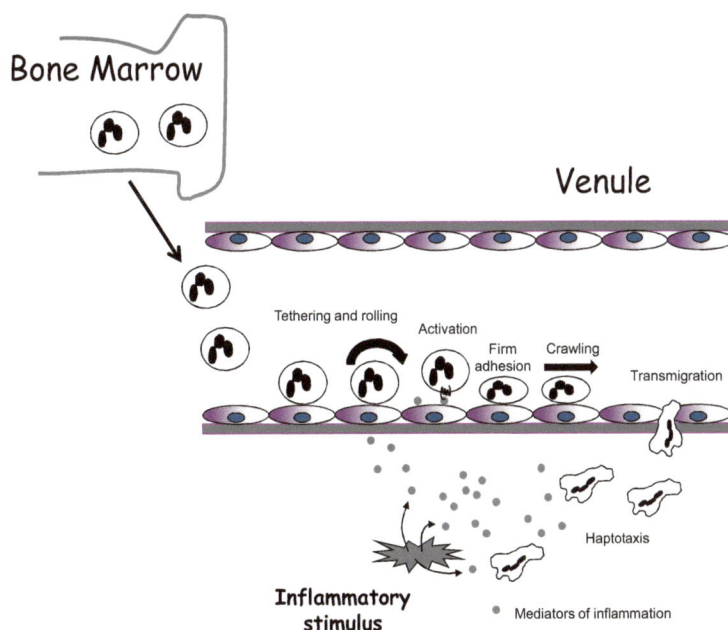

Figure 1: Paradigm for neutrophil recruitment into sites of inflammation. Neutrophils are produced in bone marrow and gain access to the circulation. In sites of inflammation, neutrophils are tethered to and roll on endothelial cells expressing selectins or

selectin ligands. Seven transmembrane receptors on the surface of rolling neutrophils may be activated by chemoattractant molecules, such as chemokines. This process leads to activation of integrins on the surface of neutrophils, binding to their ligands on endothelial cells and firm adhesion. Adherent neutrophils crawl to areas where they may transmigrate through the endothelial cell barrier and gain access to the tissue. In tissue, neutrophils migrate to site of infection obeying a chemical gradient which is most likely formed by molecules attached to matrix (haptotaxis).

Transient rolling helps neutrophils to probe for chemotactic factors, such as IL-8 and PAF, which are exposed on the endothelial surface and for which neutrophils have receptors. The paradigm is that neutrophils need to be **activated by chemoattractant molecules** which act on their seven transmembrane G protein-coupled receptors on the surface of neutrophils. This interaction leads to activation of G proteins and stimulates neutrophils to rapidly upregulate and increase the avidity of β_2-integrins. β_2-integrins are the most important integrins for neutrophil adhesion and include LFA-1 (lymphocyte function-associated antigen 1, also known as $\alpha_L\beta_2$-integrin or CD11a/CD18) and Mac-1 (macrophage receptor 1, also known as $\alpha_M\beta_2$-integrin or CD11b/CD18) [35]. Neutrophil integrins then bind to members of the immunoglobulin superfamily present on the surface of endothelial cells, specially ICAM-1 (intercellular adhesion molecule-1, CD54) [36], and mediate **firm adhesion** of neutrophils to endothelial cells. The importance of β_2-integrin members for neutrophil adhesion and consequent migration became evident from studies of patients with leukocyte adhesion deficiency type 1 syndrome (LAD-1). These patients have decreased life span. Clinically, disease is expressed as recurrent and severe bacterial infections in the absence of neutrophil migration into tissues, despite their very elevated levels in blood. Absence of neutrophil migration is explained by a mutation in the CD18 gene that leads to absence or aberrant synthesis of the β_2-integrin subunit, thus altering adhesion and subsequent migration of neutrophils into inflamed areas [37,38].

Following adherence, neutrophils must negotiate their transmigration into tissues through endothelial cells. This process involves platelet/endothelial cell adhesion molecule 1 (PECAM-1 or CD31), junctional adhesion molecules and CD99. More recent studies suggest that transmigration of neutrophils across the endothelium occurs more frequently at paracellular routes in discrete hot spots [39,40]. Neutrophils need to crawl to these hot spots before their transmigration into tissues. Once in tissues, neutrophils will migrate to the site of infection in response to a chemical gradient, most likely formed by chemoattractant molecules, such as chemokines, attached to the matrix, a process referred to as haptotaxis [41].

Specificity of the migration of particular leukocytes subsets is mostly specified by the set of chemoattractants expressed on tissues and the set of chemoattractant receptors expressed on the leukocyte. Many classical chemotactic factors, such as complement factor 5a (C5a), leukotriene B$_4$ (LTB$_4$), platelet-activating factor (PAF) and bacterial formyl-peptides (fMLP), activate neutrophils but are not selective for this subset of leukocytes [42]. Members of the chemokine family are thought to provide the necessary specificity for leukocyte subset migration *in vivo* [43]. CXCR1 and CXCR2 are thought to be the most relevant and active chemokine receptors expressed on neutrophils [44]. These receptors bind to a range of CXC chemokines which have an ELR+ motif, including Interleukin-8 (CXCL8). In rodents, CXCR2 appears to be more relevant for neutrophil influx but the CXCR1 receptor has been demonstrated in mice [45]. The relevance of these receptors for neutrophil influx can be demonstrated by studies showing that blockade or absence of CXCR1/2 prevented neutrophil influx in several models of disease [46]. In the context of bacterial infection, blockade of CXCR2 was associated with decreased local clearance and enhanced systemic spreading of bacteria [47-50]. Therefore, it appears that production of CXC ELR+ chemokines, including CXCL1, CXCL2 and CXCL8, and activation of their CXCR1/2 receptors is necessary for adequate migration of neutrophils in many models of disease and during bacterial infection. However, when high levels of chemokines, such as CXCL8, reach the circulation, there can be systemic activation of neutrophils, leading to their trapping of activated cells in target organs, including the lung. There may also be down regulation of CXCR1 and CXCR2 receptors, which may prevent subsequent migration of leukocytes into tissues. In this context, neutrophils isolated from septic patients demonstrate decreased chemotaxis toward IL-8 [20] and depressed expression of CXCR2 [51,52].

Once neutrophils reach the site of infection, they will interact and may phagocytose and kill bacteria. Neutrophil binding of bacteria is greatly augmented when the pathogens are coated with IgG. The high affinity receptor for IgG is CD64, which is absent from resting neutrophils and is considered to be a marker of activated neutrophils [53]. Most neutrophils from patients with sepsis express CD64 [54], and an upregulation of CD64 on neonatal neutrophils is regarded as an indicator of sepsis [55]. An increased expression of CD64 is associated with augmented respiratory burst activity [56] and this molecule is present on most neutrophils that bind to cultured endothelium, an interaction that is prevented by anti-CD64 antibodies [57]. Binding to bacteria also occurs via CD14, the co-receptor for LPS that is present on all monocytes. This receptor is weakly expressed in neutrophils but becomes upregulated in response to bacterial infection [58]. Other receptors that enhance phagocytosis and bacterial recognition include C3b receptor [59], which binds complement peptide C3b; CD16 and CD32, which like CD64 also bind the Fc sites (tail regions) of IgG. All of these receptors are adequately expressed on neutrophils from patients with sepsis [4].

Stimulated neutrophils produce ROS (reactive oxygen species) and RNS (reactive nitrogen species) through the nicotinamide adenine dinucleotide phosphate oxidase complex, myeloperoxidase and xanthine oxidoreductase and represent a defense mechanism against invading microorganisms [60]. LPS and other proinflammatory mediators activate nicotinamide adenine dinucleotide phosphate oxidase to produce superoxide radical (O^{2-}). In aqueous environments, superoxide radical is rapidly catalyzed by superoxide dismutase into hydrogen peroxide (H2O2) and hydroxyl radicals. Myeloperoxidase from neutrophil azurophilic granules produces hypochlorous acid from hydrogen peroxide (H2O2) and chloride anion (Cl-) during respiratory burst. Moreover, O^{2-} in the presence of nitric oxide, generates peroxynitrite (ONOO-). These radicals are highly cytotoxic, and neutrophils use them to kill bacteria and other pathogens [60]. Despite their importance as defense mechanism against invading pathogens, overwhelming production of ROS and RNS or deficit in oxidant scavenger and antioxidant defenses results in oxidative/nitrosative stress, a key element in the deleterious processes of sepsis [61, 62].

DYSREGULATED NEUTROPHIL MIGRATION IN SEPSIS

As argued above, neutrophil migration occurs and is necessary for the host to deal with bacterial infection in experimental models of infection. In humans, deficient neutrophil function is clearly linked to increased frequency and severity of bacterial and fungal infections [63]. Moreover, patients with low neutrophil levels, such as after chemotherapy, have increased risk for bacterial and certain fungal infections [64,65]. What is the evidence that neutrophil migration is deficient and may contribute to sepsis? It has been shown that neutrophils from septic patients exhibited an impaired chemotaxis to several chemotactic factors *in vitro*, such as fMLP, LTB₄ and CXCL-8 [20, 52, 66]. In these studies, the degree of suppression on neutrophil chemotaxis was associated with the severity of disease, suggesting that an impairment of neutrophil migration is a poor prognostic marker of this disease [20, 52, 66]. On the other hand, it has been shown that patients who suffered traumatic injury were at increased risk for the development of multisystem organ failure, and neutrophils recovered from such patients demonstrate increased chemotactic responses to CXC [66]. Furthermore, enhanced CXCR2 function has been shown to correlate with the development of organ injury, i.e., acute respiratory distress syndrome, whereas decreased function correlated to predisposition to pneumonia and sepsis [66, 67]. It is clear from these studies that neutrophils have to function adequately in response to infection and that excessive or blunted response may have consequences to the host. The difficulty lies in attempting to define what an appropriate response is.

If, as demonstrated above, neutrophil migration may be deficient in sepsis, the understanding of mechanisms which regulate neutrophil migration in sepsis and other pathological conditions may unravel novel strategies to control this devastating condition. We will now discuss molecular mechanisms shown to disturb neutrophil migration in experimental models of sepsis.

MECHANISMS OF THE IMPAIRMENT OF NEUTROPHIL MIGRATION IN SEPSIS

Studies investigating mechanisms by which sepsis leads to impairment of neutrophil migration and the relevance of this phenomenon for the outcome of sepsis have been mostly carried out in rodents, especially in models of sepsis caused by cecal ligation and puncture (CLP). In these studies, failure of neutrophil migration was associated with increased number of bacteria in peritoneal exudates and blood, followed by systemic inflammation and reduction in survival rate [21] (Fig. **2**). The systemic inflammatory response was characterized by increased levels of circulating cytokines and chemokines and neutrophil sequestration in the lung [21]. This is similar to findings in patients, as described above. In our studies, failure of neutrophil migration was not a consequence of chemotactic mediator loss, as there were elevated levels of chemotactic mediators at the infection site [19, 68]. Indeed, levels of chemotactic mediators were greater than those found in sites of bacterial infection in which control of infection was attained [19, 68]. *In vitro* studies demonstrate that neutrophil movement (chemotaxis) in response to chemoattractants was deficient, suggesting a neutrophil-intrinsic defect in response to chemoattractant molecules. In addition to a neutrophil-intrinsic defect, intravital microscopic studies showed decreased rolling and adhesion of neutrophils on mesenteric endothelium of animals undergoing severe CLP [69]. The latter studies suggest that alterations in neutrophil-endothelial cell interactions may also be implicated in the impairment of neutrophil migration. Although the precise mechanisms involved in the failure of neutrophils to migrate in the context of severe sepsis are not completely understood, several molecules and molecular pathways have been implicated in this phenomenon (Fig. 3). These are discussed in detail below.

Nitric oxide (NO) is a hydrophobic free radical that promptly diffuses across biological membranes. NO is produced from L-arginine and oxygen in a reaction catalyzed by a family of enzymes: NO synthases (NOS).

Three isoforms of this enzyme have been identified, namely neuronal (nNOS or type I), inducible (iNOS or type II), and endothelial (eNOS or type III). Type I and III are constitutively expressed isoforms, whereas type II or iNOS can be induced during immune and inflammatory responses by bacterial LPS and cytokines, including TNF-α, IL-1β, interferon (IFN)-α, β and γ, and chemokines [70]. Pharmacological inhibition of NOS or genetic deficiency of NOS gene enhances the migration of neutrophil into the inflammatory site in response to several stimuli [69, 71, 72]. The mechanisms by which NO attenuates neutrophil accumulation are not fully elucidated, although evidence suggest that NO, released by either eNOS or iNOS modulates leukocyte–endothelial cell interactions. Selective inhibitors of both iNOS and eNOS increase neutrophil adhesion to endothelial cells, while NO donors decrease both adhesion and leukocyte transmigration to inflammatory sites [73, 74]. These parameters are also increased in iNOS-deficient mice (iNOS-/-) [75]. The expression of cell adhesion molecules such as CD11b/CD18, L-, P- and E-selectins, ICAM-1, and VCAM-1 are down-regulated by NO donors and up-regulated by NOS inhibitors [73, 76]. In addition, complementary studies have demonstrated the participation of ICAM-1 in down-modulating the effect of NO released during inflammation on the adhesion and transmigration of neutrophils.

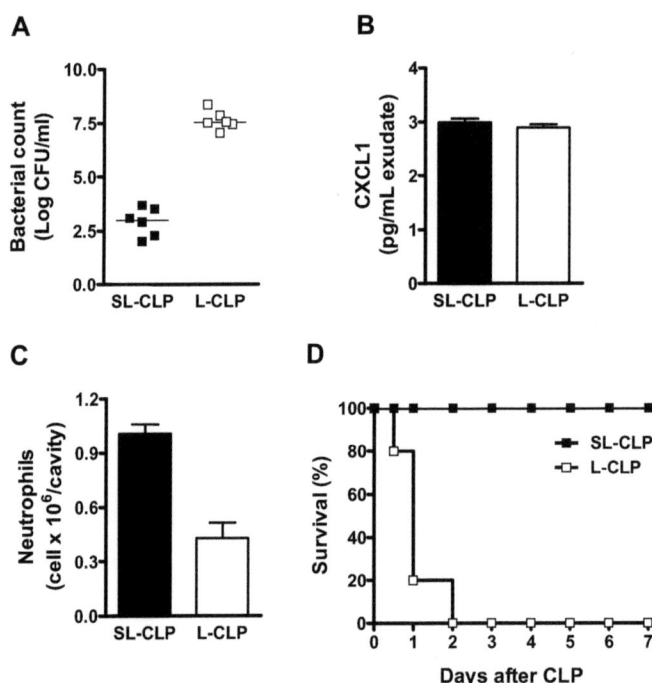

Figure 2: Failure of neutrophil migration in an experimental model of sepsis. In a model of cecal ligation and puncture (CLP), multiple punctures of the cecum with large bore needles will cause massive local infection (A), as determined by the high number of bacteria in the peritoneal fluid, whereas less punctures or use of smaller bore needles will cause extravasation of less bacteria. Despite the large number of bacteria and the (B) increased production of chemoattractant molecules (in this case, the chemokine CXCL1) observed in severe CLP, there is (C) failure of neutrophils to migrate to the site of infection. Note that number of neutrophils is greater in mild CLP, despite decreased bacterial load and local production of chemoattractant molecules. (D) The consequence of decreased neutrophil migration is the greater lethality rates observed in severe CLP.

These effects are dependent on cyclic guanosine monophosphate (cGMP) [77], a product of NO activated soluble guanylate cyclase [78], as inhibitors of guanylate cyclase prevent the inhibitory effects of NO donors on the adhesion of leukocytes, as well as on the expression of adhesion molecules [76]. In the context of sepsis, neutrophil paralysis and reduction of rolling/adhesion found in lethal sepsis were not observed in iNOS-deficient mice or in animals treated with aminoguanidine, a selective iNOS inhibitor [69, 71, 72]. Attempts to block the production of NO in clinical sepsis were conceived via an assumption that NO upregulation is maladaptive. One randomized controlled trial of nonspecific iNOS blockade was halted early when interim analysis demonstrated increased mortality in the iNOS blockade group [79]. One possibility to explain these results derives from the relevance of NO-dependent killing in the control of infection that causes sepsis [75].

Excessive production of cytokines and chemokines at the site of infection may lead to enhanced concentration of these molecules in the circulation and contribute to the failure of neutrophils to migrate in the context of severe sepsis. This role of cytokines and chemokines in severe sepsis is based on several lines of evidence. Indeed, concentration of circulating cytokines and chemokines are significantly increased in septic patients [80, 81] and in animals subjected to lethal sepsis [19, 82-84]. In neonatal sepsis, massive fresh plasma transfusion was able to restore deficiency in neutrophil chemotactic function [85], reinforcing the idea that it is the systemic levels of cytokines that associates with impairment of migration. Consistently with the latter possibility, intravenous administration of IL-2, TNF-α or CXCL-8 inhibited neutrophil migration induced by different inflammatory stimuli [84, 86-88]. Interestingly, the ability of cytokines to induce impairment of neutrophil migration to sites of inflammation was blunted in the absence or after inhibition of NO production [84, 86-88]. The relevance of TNF-α for impairment of neutrophil migration was shown in TNFR1/R2-deficient mice, which survive lethal polymicrobial infection with enhanced neutrophil recruitment and bacterial clearance in the peritoneal cavity [89]. Altogether, these data suggest that an overproduction of cytokines and chemokines drive NO production in lethal sepsis and these are critical events which contribute to the impairment of neutrophil migration to the infection site [21]. Mechanistically, NO functions as a result of reduction in neutrophil/endothelium adhesion and chemotaxis.

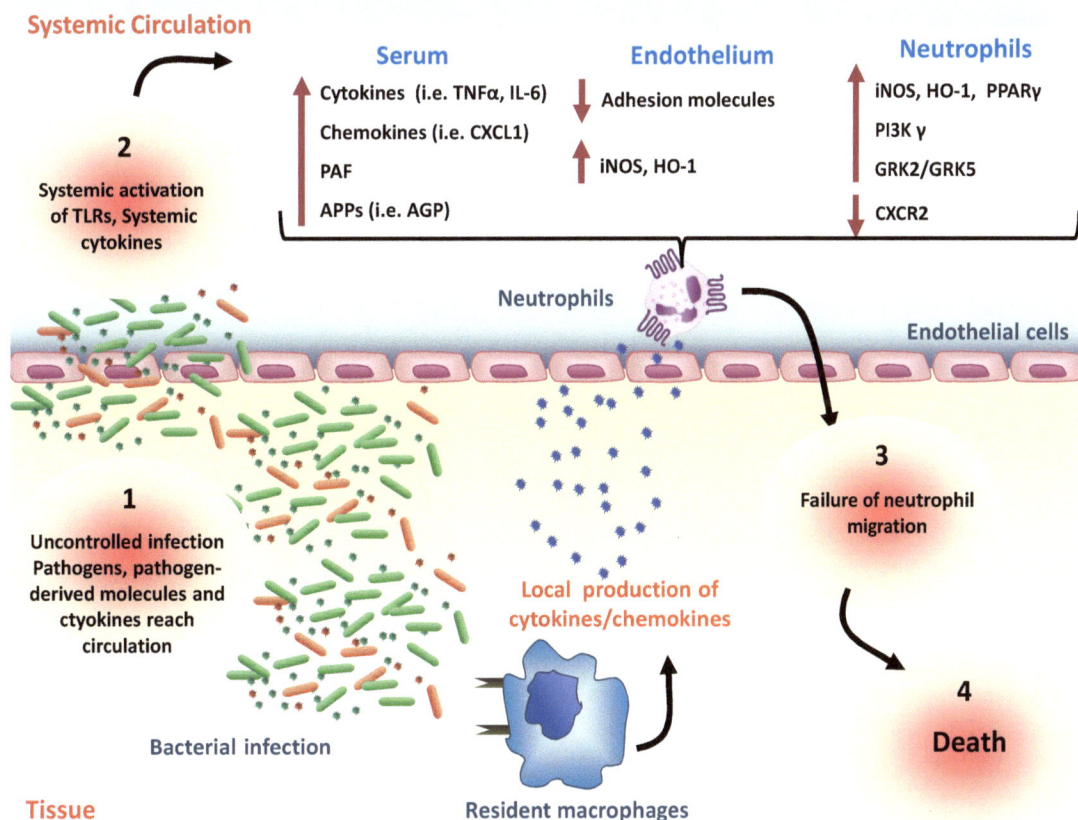

Figure 3: Molecular pathways associated with the failure of neutrophils to migrate in experimental sepsis. Several molecular pathways contribute to the failure of neutrophils to migrate in severe sepsis. See the text for detailed contribution of each pathway.

Consistent evidence has demonstrated that several deleterious effects attributed to NO, are, in fact, mediated by **ONOO-** [90]. It is well known, for example, that NO interacts with superoxide anion (O2∑-), a reactive oxygen radical forming peroxynitrite (ONOO-), a strong oxidizing agent, that can initiate lipid peroxidation, protein oxidation and nitration of tyrosine residues. These post translational modifications result in enzyme and receptor inactivation [91-94]. In this context, our laboratory demonstrated that a reduction of neutrophil/endothelium cell interaction, and consequently the failure of neutrophil migration observed in CLP-induced severe sepsis were partially mediated by ONOO- [95]. It was observed that pretreatment of septic mice with uric acid (UA) or with Tetrakis, both ONOO- scavengers, improved neutrophil rolling, adhesion and migration to the infection focus and as a consequence, decreased bacterial counts in the circulation [96]. In addition, a reduced systemic inflammatory response determined by circulating cytokine levels and neutrophil sequestration into lung tissue was observed, and consequently an improvement in survival rate. Moreover, UA pretreatment blocked the inhibitory effect of SIN-1 (an ONOO- donor) upon leukocyte rolling, adhesion and migration but was ineffective against SNAP (a specific NO donor). These results, apart from confirming that UA inactivates ONOO-, suggest that NO is able to inhibit neutrophil migration by mechanism(s) independent of ONOO- formation. It has been demonstrated that ONOO- may reduce leukocyte chemotactic activity by causing nitration of tyrosine residues on neutrophils, thereby inhibiting actin polymerization [97]. Peroxynitrite may also decrease leukocyte-endothelium interactions [95], via down regulation of P-selectin adhesion molecule expression on endothelial cells [98]. Therefore, in the context of sepsis, ONOO- generation, in addition to NO generation, partially mediates the failure of neutrophil migration into infection sites and, hence, susceptibility to severe sepsis.

Systemic inflammatory response results in elevation of the concentration of **acute-phase proteins (APP)** in plasma, and these proteins can contribute to neutrophil migration failure in severe sepsis. Recently, we isolated and identified alpha-1-acid glycoprotein (AGP) from the serum of severe septic patients. Both the isolated protein and a commercial sample of AGP inhibited carrageenan-induced neutrophil migration into the peritoneal cavity of rats when given intravenously. Analysis by intravital microscopy demonstrated that both proteins inhibited rolling and adhesion of leukocytes in the mesenteric microcirculation. Interestingly, the inhibitory effect was blocked by aminoguanidine, a NOS inhibitor, and was not observed in iNOS knockout mice. Moreover, neutrophils from healthy subjects incubated with AGP had increased (~2.5-fold) nitrite content in the supernatant. In agreement with this, the administration of AGP to rats with mild CLP sepsis inhibited neutrophil migration and reduced 7-day survival from ~80% to 20%. These data demonstrate that AGP inhibits neutrophil migration by an NO-dependent process [99]. AGP may also bind to negatively charged sialyl Lewis X residues on the surface of neutrophils, hence inhibiting selectin-Lewis X interactions between membranes of neutrophils and endothelial cells [100]. The concentration of AGP is greatly increased in the serum of septic patients [101], suggesting that, akin to cytokines, AGP may also contribute to inhibition of neutrophil migration in human sepsis.

Numerous studies have demonstrated that **heme oxygenase** (HO), a microsomal enzyme that catalyzes the degradation of heme into carbon monoxide (CO), biliverdin (BVD) and free iron [102], as well as its end products are able to modulate the inflammatory process [103, 104]. Three HO isoforms have been characterized. HO-1, an inducible isoform, is expressed in a variety of cells including endothelial, vascular smooth cells, basophils, monocytes/macrophages and neutrophils. HO-1 expression can be modulated by cytokines, NO, endotoxin, heme and during an inflammatory response [104-111]. HO-2 and HO-3 are isoforms constitutively expressed in brain, testis and endothelium [112, 113]. There is evidence that NO derived from iNOS induces HO-1 expression [114] and potentiates HO-1 induction by ferriprotoporfyrin IX chloride (hemin) [115]. Our group has shown that HO-1 metabolites (biliverdin and CO) inhibit neutrophil migration into the site of inflammation by reducing neutrophil rolling and adhesion [111] and there is evidence that **bilirubin and CO levels** are respectively elevated in serum and in exhaled breath of patients with severe sepsis [116, 117], suggesting that the HO-1 pathway has a potential role in the pathogenesis of sepsis. Studies on the role of HO-1 in sepsis have been conducted in our laboratory. We found that there is an increased expression of HO-1 in mesenteric tissue and in circulating neutrophils of mice undergoing CLP. Importantly, pharmacological inhibition of HO-1 restored the endothelium-leukocyte interaction and the migration of neutrophil into the infection site, indicating that HO-1 plays a role in the failure of neutrophil migration to infection focus in severe sepsis (our unpublished data).

The **peroxisome proliferator activated receptor gamma** (PPARγ) is a member in the nuclear receptor superfamily which mediates part of the regulatory effects of dietary fatty acids on gene expression. More recently, PPARγ has been recognized as playing an important role as a negative regulator of neutrophil migration. Treatment with either the synthetic PPARγ agonists (troglitazone or rosiglitazone) or the natural agonist 15-deoxy-delta-12,14-prostaglandin J2 (15d-PGJ2) inhibited neutrophil chemotaxis in response to IL-8 or fMLP (Napimoga, Vieira *et al.* 2008; Reddy, Narala *et al.* 2008). Moreover, we have shown that treatment with 15d-PGJ2 inhibited neutrophil rolling and adherence to endothelium by suppressing the ICAM-1 expression on endothelium, an NO-dependent mechanism [118]. Importantly, increased expression of PPARγ was found in neutrophils isolated either from septic mice or from sepsis patients [119].

Toll-like receptors (TLRs) are germ line-encoded pattern recognition receptors, and more than 11 members have been identified. Several TLRs recognize different bacterial products: TLR2 recognizes specific components of Mycobacterium spp. (lipoarabinomannan), fungi (zymosan), and gram-positive bacteria (lipoteichoic acid, lipoproteins); TLR4 recognizes endotoxin or lipopolysaccharide (LPS) [120, 121]; TLR5 recognizes and is activated by bacterial flagellin; and TLR9 recognizes unmethylated DNA containing CpG motifs [122]. Although TLRs are essential components of the innate immune response to infection, a growing body of evidence indicates that these receptors may also play a role in the pathophysiology of sepsis [123-125]. Accordingly, many groups have clearly demonstrated that deficiency or blockade of TLRs protects mice from experimental models of sepsis [68, 126-129]. Investigating the harmful role of TLRs during polymicrobial sepsis, we demonstrated that systemic activation of TLR2 and TLR4 impaired the migration of neutrophils into the site of infection by down-regulating the expression of the chemokine receptor CXCR2 in circulating neutrophils [68, 127].

The **chemokine receptor CXCR2** is highly expressed in neutrophils and, as discussed above, signaling through this receptor is essential for the maximal recruitment of the neutrophil into the inflammatory site [130]. Decreased expression of CXCR2 has been observed in neutrophils isolated from sepsis patients [51, 52]. In experimental sepsis, the expression of CXCR2 on neutrophils from mice undergoing severe sepsis was significantly reduced when compared to neutrophils from mice undergoing mild sepsis or sham-operation. The reduction of CXCR2 was re-established by genetic inhibition of TLR2 or TLR4 [68, 127], as well as by pharmacological and genetic inhibition of iNOS [50]. Moreover, inhibitors of iNOS prevented TLR agonists-induced CXCR2 down-regulation in neutrophils, and, the NO donor, SNAP, inhibited CXCL8-induced human neutrophil chemotaxis and CXCR2 expression on both human and murine neutrophils [50, 88]. These results highlight that the excessive production of NO during sepsis induced by Toll-like activation reduces the expression of CXCR2 on the neutrophil surface and contributes to the failure of neutrophil migration [50].

A large number of inflammatory mediators are involved in neutrophil recruitment [131]. Independent of the chemical nature of the chemoattractant, most of them exert their action via binding to G protein-coupled receptors (GPCRs) [132]. The activation of these chemotactic receptors triggers a complex cascade of signaling events; activating tyrosine kinase. This is a key event in mediating actin filament assembly and a fundamental step for cell locomotion [132-134]. Most GPCRs display a rapid loss of responsiveness in the continuing presence of chemoattractants, in a process of desensitization that involves the phosphorylation of agonist-occupied GPCR by **GPCR kinase** (GRK) [135]. Therefore, a continuous and excessive activation of chemokine receptors can induce an increase in the expression of GRKs, which phosphorylate GPCRs and thereby instigate signal receptor desensitization [136]. A relationship between altered GPCR signaling and changes in the expression of GRKs has been clearly demonstrated [135]. Taking these findings in account, we investigated whether the activation of GRKs is involved in the desensitization of CXCR2 in neutrophils from septic patients and mice undergoing severe sepsis. We have observed that neutrophils from septic patients and animals, in comparison with control neutrophils, showed an increased expression of GRK2 and GRK5 [127, 137]. Similarly, pretreatment of cells from healthy controls with cytokines or LPS induced up-regulation of GRK2 expression in neutrophils [137]. These data suggest that high systemic levels of inflammatory mediators or TLRs agonists in sepsis could over-stimulate circulating neutrophils, inducing GRK expression and GPCR phosphorylation. Thus, desensitization of GPCR which is most probably induced by the overproduction of mediators or circulating microorganism byproducts in severe septic patients may account for the unresponsiveness of neutrophils to chemoattractants during sepsis.

The molecular mechanisms associated with GRK expression and GPCR phosphorylation remain not elucidated, but we recently proposed that PI3K/AKT pathway might be involved in this process. **Phosphoinositide-3 kinases (PI3Ks)** are intracellular signaling enzymes involved in various aspects of septic pathophysiology, including inflammatory cell recruitment and activation [138], apoptosis [139], and coagulation [140]. Through these actions, PI3Ks contribute to organ dysfunction, including that of the lung [141], liver [142] and cardiovascular system [143], each susceptible to septic injury. Unlike other isoforms, PI3Kγ is activated by the βγ subunit of GPCRs to produce the second messenger PIP3 [144]. PIP3 subsequently acts as a docking site for Akt/PKB and PDK1, which in turn phosphorylate various cellular molecules inducing biological effects such as proliferation, differentiation and survival [144]. In murine sepsis model, both genetic absence or pharmacological inhibition of PI3Kγ kinase significantly improved survival, reduced multi-organ damage and limited bacterial decompartmentalization. Protection resulted, at least in part, from neutrophil-dependent mechanisms. Indeed, absence of PI3Kγ function prevented the failure of neutrophils to migrate during severe sepsis by maintaining surface expression of CXCR2 on the surface of neutrophils. Furthermore, inhibition of PI3Kγ with a selective inhibitor significantly decreased mortality, improved neutrophil migration and bacterial control, even when the drug was administered during established septic shock [145]. These results are in agreement with the notion that desensitization of GPCRs, such as CXCR2, depends on PI3Kγ kinase activity. Moreover, these studies highlight the potential therapeutic benefits of blocking PI3Kγ in the context of human sepsis, a possibility that will have to be investigated in appropriate clinical trials.

IL-33 is a recently identified member of the IL-1 family that binds the heterodimeric receptor complex consisting of ST2 (IL-1RL1) and the IL-1 receptor accessory protein [146-148]. ST2 is mainly expressed on T_H2 cells and mast cells and has a key role in T_H2 effector functions [149,150]. Moreover, ST2 can negatively regulate TLR activation via sequestration of the TLR signaling components myeloid differentiation factor-88 (MyD88) and Mal [151, 152]. In a recent study, it was demonstrated that IL-33 activated neutrophils, preventing the induction of GRK2 mediated by TLR signaling. This was associated with maintenance of the expression of CXCR2 on the surface of neutrophils, thus empowering their migration to the site of infection. By preventing the failure of neutrophil migration during sepsis, IL-33 reduced the sequestration of neutrophils in the lungs and improved survival, suggesting IL-33 may have therapeutic potential in sepsis and may be an important endogenous regulator of the impairment of neutrophil migration [153].

Another study highlighted the importance of **platelet-activating factor** (PAF) as a negative regulator of neutrophil migration [154]. PAF is a potent phospholipid mediator synthesized by a large number of cells, including platelets, endothelial cells, macrophage, and neutrophils [155, 156]. Its biological activity is mediated through a G protein-linked receptor (PAFR) that is expressed on the surface of a variety of cell types [155-157] and regulated through a rapid degradation by PAF-acetylhydrolase [158-159]. It was shown that inhibition of PAFR signaling, using a PAFR antagonist or PAFR-deficient mice, provided significant protection from CLP-induced mortality in lethal sepsis, which was associated with an enhancement of neutrophil migration into the infectious site and improvement of bacterial clearance [154]. This study suggests that PAF may be one of the mechanisms contributing to the impaired migration observed in severe sepsis. Further studies are necessary to understand how activation of PAFR interacts with CXCR2 and the PI3Kγ pathway.

Altogether these studies suggest that several molecules and pathways contribute to the failure of neutrophils to migrate into sites infection during severe sepsis (Fig. **3**). Mediators of inflammation and signaling pathways often interact to induce optimal recruitment of leukocytes *in vivo* [160, 161]. In the context of sepsis, there is overwhelming production of many mediators of inflammation and it is likely that these same molecules and pathways may interact to prevent adequate immune function and, in the context of the present discussion, neutrophil migration (Fig. **3**).

THE CONSEQUENCE OF FAILURE OF NEUTROPHILS TO MIGRATE: MULTI-ORGAN FAILURE

As mentioned above, failure of neutrophils to migrate into sites of infection is a hallmark of and contributing factor to severe sepsis. In sepsis, neutrophils engage in repelling invading pathogens while simultaneously inducing collateral damage in which organ function is the casualty. As in most inflammatory reactions, there is a considerable reserve pool of mature neutrophils within the bone marrow which is rapidly mobilized in the early phase of sepsis. However, in severe sepsis, this mobilization of neutrophils occurs in the absence of their migration to sites of infection and in presence of large quantities of cytokines and other molecules in the circulation. This combination of large numbers of neutrophils, sometimes with large quantities of immature neutrophils, and molecules which can prime or activate neutrophils sets the scene for injury to multiple organs.

The diagnostic criteria for sepsis include leukocytosis, leukopenia or normal white blood cell count with more than 10% of immature cells [162]. This variation probably reflects different stages and severity of sepsis. As reasoned above, presence of large number of circulating neutrophils could be detrimental in sepsis. However, it is more likely that it is not the presence of neutrophils in blood that matters, but their entrapment in target organs, such as the lung, liver and kidney. Indeed, the finding that neutrophil-mediated lung injury may occur in patients with neutropenia [163] suggests that organ dysfunction might be initiated by only a few neutrophils sequestered in the microvasculature. Alternatively, the low number in the circulation could be secondary to the high number of neutrophils entrapped and causing damage to the lung. It must be noted that electron microscopy studies have shown that neutrophils do not necessarily migrate into the lung tissue during non-pulmonary sepsis but become entrapped in the microcirculation [164]. In addition, it is possible that presence of a subset of neutrophils whose phenotype and level of activation favors induction of tissue damage [165] may occur and contribute to the pathogenesis of sepsis. In animal models of sepsis, immature neutrophils preferentially accumulate in pulmonary microvessels in which their activation induces substantial tissue damage [166].

But why do neutrophils become entrapped in the lung and other organs? In the systemic circulation, neutrophils enter tissues via postcapillary venules via a process that needs rolling and subsequent adhesion (see above and Fig. **1**). In the pulmonary circulation, emigration occurs via the capillaries and the paradigm for migration is significantly different. The lumen of pulmonary capillaries (7-10 um) is so narrow that neutrophils (10-15 um) need to negotiate their passage through the lungs each time. This close contact of neutrophils and the pulmonary microcirculation extends neutrophil transit time and prevents rolling along the endothelium. In the context of systemic inflammation, neutrophils are activated in the circulation and become stiff (rigid), markedly enhancing their transit time through the lungs [167]. The combination of an activated neutrophil with enhanced transit time may cause lung damage [168-171]. Recent studies have suggested that similar mechanisms may lead to entrapment of neutrophils in hepatic sinusoids [172]. It has been suggested that platelet-neutrophil interactions may actually facilitate the entrapment of neutrophils in the liver [173].

While it was previously assumed that the sequestration of primed neutrophils could be a key stage in the initiation of multiple organ failure, a second "activation" step is essential for tissue damage to occur [164]. Different conditions associated with systemic neutrophil priming cause retention of neutrophils in the lung but often no injury. It is possible that many neutrophils primed in the circulation, for example, in the context of systemic vasculitis, major burns, and pancreatitis, become trapped in the pulmonary microcirculation, and if not induced to migrate by a secondary stimulus (e.g., infection) can "de-prime" and be released back into the circulating pool in a quiescent state [174]. It is of note that most severe septic patients are under mechanical ventilation and may be exposed to secondary pulmonary infection.

In addition to causing damage by interacting with the microvasculature of various organs, neutrophils may also interact with the coagulation system in localized inflammation and in generalized sepsis. During systemic inflammation, homeostatic mechanisms are compromised in the microcirculation including endothelial hyperactivity, fibrin deposition, microvascular occlusion, and cellular exudates that further impede adequate tissue oxygenation. Neutrophils participate in these rheologic changes through their augmented binding to blood vessel walls and through the formation of platelet-leukocyte aggregates [175]. Neutrophil elastase, other proteases, glycases and inflammatory cytokines degrade endogenous anticoagulant activity, and impair fibrinolysis on endothelial surfaces favouring a procoagulant state [176]. Intensive care unit patients, especially severe septic ones, are at risk of deep venous thrombosis (DVT) and pulmonary embolism, and must receive DVT prophylaxis with either a low dose unfractionated heparin or low-molecular weight heparin unless there are contraindications (i.e., thrombocytopenia, severe coagulopathy, active bleeding, recent intracerebral hemorrhage) [1].

CONCLUDING REMARKS

The discussion above highlights the potential participation of neutrophils in sepsis, with particular emphasis on the relevance of the mechanisms and relevance of the failure of neutrophil migration to the outcome of sepsis. Mediators of inflammation are released in response to infection and are important for the migration of neutrophils to the site of infection, where neutrophils will interact and deal with the infecting microbe (Fig. **1**). However, these same mediators which are relevant for neutrophil influx may reach or be produced in the circulation and cause a systemic inflammatory response. This systemic inflammation is associated with activation of key signaling pathways in neutrophils, including activation of PI3Kγ and GRK2, loss of CXCR2 expression and failure of neutrophils to migrate. Decreased neutrophil migration will mean enhanced bacterial proliferation and enhanced number of activated neutrophils in the circulation. Tissue damage and multi-organ failure may ensue. Understanding in detail mechanisms which mediate failure of neutrophils to migrate to the infection focus and mechanisms of enhanced activation of neutrophils in the circulation may unravel novel therapeutic opportunities for the treatment of sepsis. The limits of animal models are obvious but these do point objectively to possible molecular mechanisms to focus on in clinical studies and drug development.

ACKNOWLEDGEMENTS

We are grateful to Fundacao de Amparo a Pesquisas do Estado de Minas Gerais (FAPEMIG, Brazil), Fundacao de Amparo a Pesquisas do Estado de São Paulo (FAPESP, Brazil) and Conselho Nacional de Desenvolvimento Cientifico e Tecnologico (CNPq, Brazil) for financial support.

REFERENCES

[1]   Balk RA. Severe sepsis and septic shock. Definitions, epidemiology, and clinical manifestations. Crit Care Clin 2000; 16: 179-92.

[2]   Levy MM, Fink MP, Marshall JC, *et al*. SCCM/ESICM/ACCP/ATS/SIS. 2001 SCCM/ESICM/ACCP/ATS/SIS International Sepsis Definitions Conference. Crit Care Med 2003; 31: 1250-6.

[3]   Brown KA, Brain SD, Pearson JD, Edgeworth JD, Lewis SM, Treacher DF. Neutrophils in development of multiple organ failure in sepsis. Lancet 2006; 368: 157-69.

[4]   Polderman KH, Girbes AR. Drug intervention trials in sepsis: divergent results. Lancet 2004; 363: 1721-3.

[5]   Singer M, De Santis V, Vitale D, Jeffcoate W. Multiorgan failure is an adaptive, endocrine-mediated, metabolic response to overwhelming systemic inflammation. Lancet 2004; 364: 545-8.

[6]   Kumar V, Sharma A. Is neuroimmunomodulation a future therapeutic approach for sepsis? Int Immunopharmacol 2010; 10: 9-17.

[7]   Cohen J. The immunopathogenesis of sepsis. Nature 2002; 420: 885-91.

[8]   Levi M, van der Poll T. Inflammation and coagulation. Crit Care Med 2010; 38: S26-34.

[9]   Sørensen TI, Nielsen GG, Andersen PK, Teasdale TW. Genetic and environmental influences on premature death in adult adoptees. N Engl J Med 1988; 318: 727-32.

[10]   Namath A, Patterson AJ. Genetic polymorphisms in sepsis. Crit Care Clin 2009; 25: 835-56.

[11]   Víctor VM, Espulgues JV, Hernández-Mijares A, Rocha M. Oxidative stress and mitochondrial dysfunction in sepsis: a potential therapy with mitochondria-targeted antioxidants. Infect Disord Drug Targets 2009; 9: 376-89.

[12]   Ruggieri AJ, Levy RJ, Deutschman CS. Mitochondrial dysfunction and resuscitation in sepsis. Crit Care Clin 2010; 26: 567-75.

[13]   Nascimento DC, Alves-Filho JC, Sônego F, *et al*. Role of regulatory T cells in long-term immune dysfunction associated with severe sepsis. Crit Care Med 2010; 38: 1718-25.

[14]   Nduka OO, Parrillo JE. The pathophysiology of septic shock. Crit Care Clin 2009; 25: 677-702.

[15]   Kerschen E, Hernandez I, Zogg M, *et al*. Activated protein C targets CD8+ dendritic cells to reduce the mortality of endotoxemia in mice. J Clin Invest 2010; 120: 3167-78.

[16]   Ait-Oufella H, Maury E, Lehoux S, Guidet B, Offenstadt G. The endothelium: physiological functions and role in microcirculatory failure during severe sepsis. Intensive Care Med 2010; 36: 1286-98.

[17]   Rahman M, Zhang S, Chew M, Ersson A, Jeppsson B, Thorlacius H. Platelet-derived CD40L (CD154) mediates neutrophil upregulation of Mac-1 and recruitment in septic lung injury. Ann Surg 2009; 250: 783-90.

[18]   Benjamim CF, Ferreira SH, Cunha FQ. Role of nitric oxide in the failure of neutrophil migration in sepsis. J Infect Dis 2000; 182: 214-23.

[19]   Tavares-Murta BM, Zaparoli M, Ferreira RB, *et al*. Failure of neutrophil chemotactic function in septic patients. Crit Care Med 2002; 30: 1056-61.

[20]   Alves-Filho JC, Spiller F, Cunha FQ. Neutrophil paralysis in sepsis. Shock 2010; 34 Suppl 1: 15-21.

[21]   Nathan C. Neutrophils and immunity: challenges and opportunities. Nat Rev Immunol 2006; 6: 173-82.

[22]   Kilpatrick LE, Standage SW, Li H, *et al*. Protection against sepsis-induced lung injury by selective inhibition of protein kinase C-{delta} ({delta}-PKC). J Leukoc Biol 2010; [Epub ahead of print].

[23]   Holman JM Jr, Saba TM. Hepatocyte injury during post-operative sepsis: activated neutrophils as potential mediators. J Leukoc Biol 1988; 43: 193-203.

[24]   Huynh T, Nguyen N, Keller S, Moore C, Shin MC, McKillop IH. Reducing leukocyte trafficking preserves hepatic function after sepsis. J Trauma 2010; 69: 360-7.

[25]   Thijs A, Thijs LG. Pathogenesis of renal failure in sepsis. Kidney Int Suppl 1998; 66: S34-7.

[26]   Gonçalves GM, Zamboni DS, Câmara NO. The role of innate immunity in septic acute kidney injuries. Shock 2010; 34 Suppl 1: 22-6.

[27]   Souto FO, Alves-Filho JC, Turato WM, Auxiliadora-Martins M, Basile-Filho A, Cunha FQ. Essential Role of CCR2 in Neutrophil Tissue Infiltration and Multiple Organ Dysfunction in Sepsis. Am J Respir Crit Care Med 2010; [Epub ahead of print].

[28]   Drost EM, Kassabian G, Meiselman HJ, Gelmont D, Fisher TC. Increased rigidity and priming of polymorphonuclear leukocytes in sepsis. Am J Respir Crit Care Med 1999; 159: 1696-702.

[29]   Skoutelis AT, Kaleridis V, Athanassiou GM, Kokkinis KI, Missirlis YF, Bassaris HP. Neutrophil deformability in patients with sepsis, septic shock, and adult respiratory distress syndrome. Crit Care Med 2000; 28: 2355-9.

[30]   Furze RC, Rankin SM. Neutrophil mobilization and clearance in the bone marrow. Immunology 2008; 125: 281-8.

[31]   Seely AJ, Pascual JL, Christou NV. Science review: Cell membrane expression (connectivity) regulates neutrophil delivery, function and clearance. Crit Care 2003; 7: 291-307.

[32]   Muller WA. Leukocyte-endothelial-cell interactions in leukocyte transmigration and the inflammatory response. Trends Immunol 2003; 24: 327-34.

[33]   Kansas GS. Selectins and their ligands: current concepts and controversies. Blood 1996; 88: 3259-87.

[34]   Huttenlocher A, Sandborg RR, Horwitz AF. Adhesion in cell migration. Curr Opin Cell Biol 1995; 7: 697-706.

[35]   Laudanna C, Kim JY, Constantin G, Butcher E. Rapid leukocyte integrin activation by chemokines. Immunol Rev 2002; 186: 37-46.

[36]   Anderson DC, Springer TA. Leukocyte adhesion deficiency: an inherited defect in the Mac-1, LFA-1, and p150,95 glycoproteins. Annu Rev Med 1987; 38: 175-94.

[37]   Smith CW, Marlin SD, Rothlein R, Toman C, Anderson DC. Cooperative interactions of LFA-1 and Mac-1 with intercellular adhesion molecule-1 in facilitating adherence and transendothelial migration of human neutrophils *in vitro*. J Clin Invest 1989; 83: 2008-17.

[38]   Phillipson M, Heit B, Colarusso P, Liu L, Ballantyne CM, Kubes P. Intraluminal crawling of neutrophils to emigration sites: a molecularly distinct process from adhesion in the recruitment cascade. J Exp Med 2006; 203: 2569-75.

[39]   Schenkel AR, Mamdouh Z, Muller WA. Locomotion of monocytes on endothelium is a critical step during extravasation. Nat Immunol 2004; 5: 393-400.

[40]   Rot A. Neutrophil attractant/activation protein-1 (interleukin-8) induces *in vitro* neutrophil migration by haptotactic mechanism. Eur J Immunol 1993; 23: 303-6.

[41]   Bokoch GM. Chemoattractant signaling and leukocyte activation. Blood 1995; 86: 1649-60.

[42]   Bonecchi R, Galliera E, Borroni EM, Corsi MM, Locati M, Mantovani A. Chemokines and chemokine receptors: an overview. Front Biosci 2009; 14: 540-51.

[43]   Stillie R, Farooq SM, Gordon JR, Stadnyk AW. The functional significance behind expressing two IL-8 receptor types on PMN. J Leukoc Biol 2009; 86: 529-43.

[44]   Fu W, Zhang Y, Zhang J, Chen WF. Cloning and characterization of mouse homolog of the CXC chemokine receptor CXCR1. Cytokine 2005; 31: 9-17.

[45]   Bizzarri C, Beccari AR, Bertini R, Cavicchia MR, Giorgini S, Allegretti M. ELR+ CXC chemokines and their receptors (CXC chemokine receptor 1 and CXC chemokine receptor 2) as new therapeutic targets. Pharmacol Ther 2006; 112: 139-49.

[46]   Olszyna DP, Florquin S, Sewnath M, *et al.* CXC chemokine receptor 2 contributes to host defense in murine urinary tract infection. J Infect Dis 2001; 184: 301-7.

[47]   Kielian T, Barry B, Hickey WF. CXC chemokine receptor-2 ligands are required for neutrophil-mediated host defense in experimental brain abscesses. J Immunol 2001; 166: 4634-43.

[48]   Khan S, Cole N, Hume EB, *et al.* The role of CXC chemokine receptor 2 in Pseudomonas aeruginosa corneal infection. J Leukoc Biol 2007; 81: 315-8.

[49]   Rios-Santos F, Alves-Filho JC, Souto FO, *et al.* Down-regulation of CXCR2 on neutrophils in severe sepsis is mediated by inducible nitric oxide synthase-derived nitric oxide. Am J Respir Crit Care Med 2007; 175: 490-7.

[50]   Cummings CJ, Martin TR, Frevert CW, *et al.* Expression and function of the chemokine receptors CXCR1 and CXCR2 in sepsis. J Immunol 1999; 162: 2341-6.

[51]   Chishti AD, Shenton BK, Kirby JA, Baudouin SV. Neutrophil chemotaxis and receptor expression in clinical septic shock. Intensive Care Med 2004; 30: 605-11.

[52]   Hoffmeyer F, Witte K, Schmidt RE. The high-affinity Fc gamma RI on PMN: regulation of expression and signal transduction. Immunology 1997; 92: 544-52.

[53]   Qureshi SS, Lewis SM, Gant VA, Treacher D, Davis BH, Brown KA. Increased distribution and expression of CD64 on blood polymorphonuclear cells from patients with the systemic inflammatory response syndrome (SIRS). Clin Exp Immunol 2001; 125: 258-65.

[54]   Layseca-Espinosa E, Pérez-González LF, Torres-Montes A, *et al.* Expression of CD64 as a potential marker of neonatal sepsis. Pediatr Allergy Immunol 2002; 13: 319-27.

[55]   Barth E, Fischer G, Schneider EM, Moldawer LL, Georgieff M, Weiss M. Peaks of endogenous G-CSF serum concentrations are followed by an increase in respiratory burst activity of granulocytes in patients with septic shock. Cytokine 2002; 17: 275-84.

[56]   Fadlon E, Vordermeier S, Pearson TC, *et al.* Blood polymorphonuclear leukocytes from the majority of sickle cell patients in the crisis phase of the disease show enhanced adhesion to vascular endothelium and increased expression of CD64. Blood 1998; 91: 266-74.

[57]   Wagner C, Deppisch R, Denefleh B, Hug F, Andrassy K, Hänsch GM. Expression patterns of the lipopolysaccharide receptor CD14, and the FCgamma receptors CD16 and CD64 on polymorphonuclear neutrophils: data from patients with severe bacterial infections and lipopolysaccharide-exposed cells. Shock 2003; 19: 5-12.

[58]   Pangburn MK, Morrison DC, Schreiber RD, Müller-Eberhard HJ. Activation of the alternative complement pathway: recognition of surface structures on activators by bound C3b. J Immunol 1980; 124: 977-82.

[59]   Fialkow L, Wang Y, Downey GP. Reactive oxygen and nitrogen species as signaling molecules regulating neutrophil function. Free Radic Biol Med 2007; 42: 153-64.

[60]   Macdonald J, Galley HF, Webster NR. Oxidative stress and gene expression in sepsis. Br J Anaesth 2003; 90: 221-32.

[61]   Matejovic M, Krouzecky A, Rokyta R Jr, *et al.* Effects of combining inducible nitric oxide synthase inhibitor and radical scavenger during porcine bacteremia. Shock 2007; 27: 61-8.

[62]   Malech HL, Gallin JI. Current concepts: immunology. Neutrophils in human diseases. N Engl J Med 1987; 317: 687-94.

[63]   Moreno García M. Neutropenia in HIV infection. An Med Interna 1997; 14: 199-208.

[64]   Lekstrom-Himes JA, Gallin JI. Immunodeficiency diseases caused by defects in phagocytes. N Engl J Med 2000; 343: 1703-14.

[65]   Tarlowe MH, Duffy A, Kannan KB, *et al.* Prospective study of neutrophil chemokine responses in trauma patients at risk for pneumonia. Am J Respir Crit Care Med 2005; 171: 753-9.

[66]   Zarbock A, Allegretti M, Ley K. Therapeutic inhibition of CXCR2 by Reparixin attenuates acute lung injury in mice. Br J Pharmacol 2008; 155: 357-64.

[67]   Alves-Filho JC, de Freitas A, Russo M, Cunha FQ. Toll-like receptor 4 signaling leads to neutrophil migration impairment in polymicrobial sepsis. Crit Care Med 2006; 34: 461-70.

[68]   Benjamim CF, Silva JS, Fortes ZB, Oliveira MA, Ferreira SH, Cunha FQ. Inhibition of leukocyte rolling by nitric oxide during sepsis leads to reduced migration of active microbicidal neutrophils. Infect Immun 2002; 70: 3602-10.

[69]   Alderton WK, Cooper CE, Knowles RG. Nitric oxide synthases: structure, function and inhibition. Biochem J 2001; 357: 593-615.

[70]   Tavares-Murta BM, Machado JS, Ferreira SH, Cunha FQ. Nitric oxide mediates the inhibition of neutrophil migration induced by systemic administration of LPS. Inflammation 2001; 25: 247-53.

[71]   Dal Secco D, Paron JA, de Oliveira SH, Ferreira SH, Silva JS, Cunha FQ. Neutrophil migration in inflammation: nitric oxide inhibits rolling, adhesion and induces apoptosis. Nitric Oxide 2003; 9: 153-64.

[72]   Lefer DJ, Jones SP, Girod WG, *et al.* Leukocyte-endothelial cell interactions in nitric oxide synthase-deficient mice. Am J Physiol 1999; 276: H1943-50.

[73]   Ialenti A, Ianaro A, Maffia P, Sautebin L, Di Rosa M. Nitric oxide inhibits leucocyte migration in carrageenin-induced rat pleurisy. Inflamm Res 2000; 49: 411-7.

[74]   Hickey MJ, Sharkey KA, Sihota EG, *et al.* Inducible nitric oxide synthase-deficient mice have enhanced leukocyte-endothelium interactions in endotoxemia. FASEB J 1997; 11: 955-64.

[75]   Kubes P, Suzuki M, Granger DN. Nitric oxide: an endogenous modulator of leukocyte adhesion. Proc Natl Acad Sci U S A 1991; 88: 4651-5.

[76]   Dal Secco D, Moreira AP, Freitas A, *et al.* Nitric oxide inhibits neutrophil migration by a mechanism dependent on ICAM-1: role of soluble guanylate cyclase. Nitric Oxide 2006; 15: 77-86.

[77]   Opal SM. The host response to endotoxin, antilipopolysaccharide strategies, and the management of severe sepsis. Int J Med Microbiol 2007; 297: 365-77.

[78]   López A, Lorente JA, Steingrub J, *et al.* Multiple-center, randomized, placebo-controlled, double-blind study of the nitric oxide synthase inhibitor 546C88: effect on survival in patients with septic shock. Crit Care Med 2004; 32: 21-30.

[79]   Ozbalkan Z, Aslar AK, Yildiz Y, Aksaray S. Investigation of the course of proinflammatory and anti-inflammatory cytokines after burn sepsis. Int J Clin Pract 2004; 58: 125-9.

[80]   ter Meulen J, Sakho M, Koulemou K, *et al.* Activation of the cytokine network and unfavorable outcome in patients with yellow fever. J Infect Dis 2004; 190: 1821-7.

[81]   Crosara-Alberto DP, Darini AL, Inoue RY, Silva JS, Ferreira SH, Cunha FQ. Involvement of NO in the failure of neutrophil migration in sepsis induced by Staphylococcus aureus. Br J Pharmacol 2002; 136: 645-58.

[82] Moreno SE, Alves-Filho JC, Alfaya TM, da Silva JS, Ferreira SH, Liew FY. IL-12, but not IL-18, is critical to neutrophil activation and resistance to polymicrobial sepsis induced by cecal ligation and puncture. J Immunol 2006; 177: 3218-24.

[83] Moreno SE, Alves-Filho JC, Bertozi G, *et al.* Systemic administration of interleukin-2 inhibits inflammatory neutrophil migration: role of nitric oxide. Br J Pharmacol 2006; 148: 1060-6.

[84] Eisenfeld L, Krause PJ, Herson VC, Block C, Schick JB, Maderazo E. Enhancement of neonatal neutrophil motility (chemotaxis) with adult fresh frozen plasma. Am J Perinatol 1992; 9: 5-8.

[85] Otsuka Y, Nagano K, Nagano K, *et al.* Inhibition of neutrophil migration by tumor necrosis factor. *Ex vivo* and *in vivo* studies in comparison with *in vitro* effect. J Immunol 1990; 145: 2639-43.

[86] Hechtman DH, Cybulsky MI, Fuchs HJ, Baker JB, Gimbrone MA Jr. Intravascular IL-8. Inhibitor of polymorphonuclear leukocyte accumulation at sites of acute inflammation. J Immunol 1991; 147: 883-92.

[87] Tavares-Murta BM, Cunha FQ, Ferreira SH. The intravenous administration of tumor necrosis factor alpha, interleukin 8 and macrophage-derived neutrophil chemotactic factor inhibits neutrophil migration by stimulating nitric oxide production. Br J Pharmacol 1998; 124: 1369-74.

[88] Secher T, Vasseur V, Poisson DM, *et al.* Crucial role of TNF receptors 1 and 2 in the control of polymicrobial sepsis. J Immunol 2009; 182: 7855-64.

[89] Smith KJ, Kapoor R, Felts PA. Demyelination: the role of reactive oxygen and nitrogen species. Brain Pathol 1999; 9: 69-92.

[90] Radi R, Beckman JS, Bush KM, Freeman BA. Peroxynitrite oxidation of sulfhydryls. The cytotoxic potential of superoxide and nitric oxide. J Biol Chem 1991; 266: 4244-50.

[91] Ischiropoulos H, Zhu L, Beckman JS. Peroxynitrite formation from macrophage-derived nitric oxide. Arch Biochem Biophys 1992; 298: 446-51.

[92] Rubbo H, Radi R, Trujillo M, *et al.* Nitric oxide regulation of superoxide and peroxynitrite-dependent lipid peroxidation. Formation of novel nitrogen-containing oxidized lipid derivatives. J Biol Chem 1994; 269: 26066-75.

[93] MacMillan-Crow LA, Crow JP, Thompson JA. Peroxynitrite-mediated inactivation of manganese superoxide dismutase involves nitration and oxidation of critical tyrosine residues. Biochemistry 1998; 37: 1613-22.

[94] Torres-Dueñas D, Celes MR, Freitas A, *et al.* Peroxynitrite mediates the failure of neutrophil migration in severe polymicrobial sepsis in mice. Br J Pharmacol 2007; 152: 341-52.

[95] Whiteman M, Halliwell B. Protection against peroxynitrite-dependent tyrosine nitration and alpha 1-antiproteinase inactivation by ascorbic acid. A comparison with other biological antioxidants. Free Radic Res 1996; 25: 275-83.

[96] Clements MK, Siemsen DW, Swain SD, *et al.* Inhibition of actin polymerization by peroxynitrite modulates neutrophil functional responses. J Leukoc Biol 2003; 73: 344-55.

[97] Lefer DJ, Scalia R, Campbell B, *et al.* Peroxynitrite inhibits leukocyte-endothelial cell interactions and protects against ischemia-reperfusion injury in rats. J Clin Invest 1997; 99: 684-91.

[98] Mestriner FL, Spiller F, Laure HJ, *et al.* Acute-phase protein alpha-1-acid glycoprotein mediates neutrophil migration failure in sepsis by a nitric oxide-dependent mechanism. Proc Natl Acad Sci USA 2007; 104: 19595-600.

[99] Fournier T, Medjoubi-N N, Porquet D. Alpha-1-acid glycoprotein. Biochim Biophys Acta 2000; 1482: 157-71.

[100] Brinkman-van der Linden EC, van Ommen EC, van Dijk W. Glycosylation of alpha 1-acid glycoprotein in septic shock: changes in degree of branching and in expression of sialyl Lewis(x) groups. Glycoconj J 1996; 13: 27-31.

[101] Abraham NG, Lin JH, Mitrione SM, Schwartzman ML, Levere RD, Shibahara S. Expression of heme oxygenase gene in rat and human liver. Biochem Biophys Res Commun 1988; 150: 717-22.

[102] Hayashi S, Takamiya R, Yamaguchi T, *et al.* Induction of heme oxygenase-1 suppresses venular leukocyte adhesion elicited by oxidative stress: role of bilirubin generated by the enzyme. Circ Res 1999; 85: 663-71.

[103] Vicente AM, Guillén MI, Habib A, Alcaraz MJ. Beneficial effects of heme oxygenase-1 up-regulation in the development of experimental inflammation induced by zymosan. J Pharmacol Exp Ther 2003; 307: 1030-7.

[104] Tenhunen R, Marver HS, Schmid R. Microsomal heme oxygenase. Characterization of the enzyme. J Biol Chem 1969; 244: 6388-94.

[105] Willis D, Moore AR, Frederick R, Willoughby DA. Heme oxygenase: a novel target for the modulation of the inflammatory response. Nat Med 1996; 2: 87-90.

[106] Terry CM, Clikeman JA, Hoidal JR, Callahan KS. Effect of tumor necrosis factor-alpha and interleukin-1 alpha on heme oxygenase-1 expression in human endothelial cells. Am J Physiol 1998; 274: H883-91.

[107] Datta PK, Lianos EA. Nitric oxide induces heme oxygenase-1 gene expression in mesangial cells. Kidney Int 1999; 55: 1734-9.

[108] Oshiro S, Takeuchi H, Matsumoto M, Kurata S. Transcriptional activation of heme oxygenase-1 gene in mouse spleen, liver and kidney cells after treatment with lipopolysaccharide or haemoglobin. Cell Biol Int 1999; 23: 465-74.

[109] Alcaraz MJ, Fernández P, Guillén MI. Anti-inflammatory actions of the heme oxygenase-1 pathway. Curr Pharm Des 2003; 9: 2541-51.

[110] Freitas A, Alves-Filho JC, Secco DD, *et al.* Heme oxygenase/carbon monoxide-biliverdin pathway down regulates neutrophil rolling, adhesion and migration in acute inflammation. Br J Pharmacol 2006; 149: 345-54.

[111] Maines MD. The heme oxygenase system: a regulator of second messenger gases. Annu Rev Pharmacol Toxicol 1997; 37: 517-54.

[112] McCoubrey WK Jr, Huang TJ, Maines MD. Isolation and characterization of a cDNA from the rat brain that encodes hemoprotein heme oxygenase-3. Eur J Biochem 1997; 247: 725-32.

[113] Vicente AM, Guillén MI, Alcaraz MJ. Modulation of haem oxygenase-1 expression by nitric oxide and leukotrienes in zymosan-activated macrophages. Br J Pharmacol 2001; 133: 920-6.

[114] Naughton P, Hoque M, Green CJ, Foresti R, Motterlini R. Interaction of heme with nitroxyl or nitric oxide amplifies heme oxygenase-1 induction: involvement of the transcription factor Nrf2. Cell Mol Biol (Noisy-le-grand) 2002; 48: 885-94.

[115] Banks JG, Foulis AK, Ledingham IM, Macsween RN. Liver function in septic shock. J Clin Pathol 1982; 35: 1249-52.

[116] Zegdi R, Perrin D, Burdin M, Boiteau R, Tenaillon A. Increased endogenous carbon monoxide production in severe sepsis. Intensive Care Med 2002; 28: 793-6.

[117] Napimoga MH, Vieira SM, Dal-Secco D, *et al.* Peroxisome proliferator-activated receptor-gamma ligand, 15-deoxy-Delta12,14-prostaglandin J2, reduces neutrophil migration via a nitric oxide pathway. J Immunol 2008; 180: 609-17.

[118] Reddy RC, Narala VR, Keshamouni VG, Milam JE, Newstead MW, Standiford TJ. Sepsis-induced inhibition of neutrophil chemotaxis is mediated by activation of peroxisome proliferator-activated receptor-{gamma}. Blood 2008; 112: 4250-8.

[119] Akira S, Takeda K. Toll-like receptor signaling. Nat Rev Immunol 2004; 4: 499-511.

[120] Akira S, Uematsu S, Takeuchi O. Pathogen recognition and innate immunity. Cell 2006; 124: 783-801.

[121] Takeda K, Akira S. Regulation of innate immune responses by Toll-like receptors. Jpn J Infect Dis 2001; 54: 209-19.

[122] Williams DL, Ha T, Li C, *et al.* Modulation of tissue Toll-like receptor 2 and 4 during the early phases of polymicrobial sepsis correlates with mortality. Crit Care Med 2003; 31: 1808-18.

[123] Ishii KJ, Akira S. Toll-like Receptors and Sepsis. Curr Infect Dis Rep 2004; 6: 361-366.

[124] Meng G, Rutz M, Schiemann M, *et al.* Antagonistic antibody prevents toll-like receptor 2-driven lethal shock-like syndromes. J Clin Invest 2004; 113: 1473-81.

[125] Plitas G, Burt BM, Nguyen HM, Bamboat ZM, DeMatteo RP. Toll-like receptor 9 inhibition reduces mortality in polymicrobial sepsis. J Exp Med 2008; 205: 1277-83.

[126] Alves-Filho JC, Freitas A, Souto FO, *et al.* Regulation of chemokine receptor by Toll-like receptor 2 is critical to neutrophil migration and resistance to polymicrobial sepsis. Proc Natl Acad Sci U S A 2009; 106: 4018-23.

[127] Andonegui G, Zhou H, Bullard D, *et al.* Mice that exclusively express TLR4 on endothelial cells can efficiently clear a lethal systemic Gram-negative bacterial infection. J Clin Invest 2009; 119: 1921-30.

[128] Roger T, Froidevaux C, Le Roy D, *et al.* Protection from lethal gram-negative bacterial sepsis by targeting Toll-like receptor 4. Proc Natl Acad Sci USA 2009; 106: 2348-52.

[129] Holmes WE, Lee J, Kuang WJ, Rice GC, Wood WI. Structure and functional expression of a human interleukin-8 receptor. Science 1991; 253: 1278-80.

[130] Baggiolini M. Chemokines and leukocyte traffic. Nature 1998; 392: 565-8.

[131] Katanaev VL. Signal transduction in neutrophil chemotaxis. Biochemistry (Mosc) 2001; 66: 351-68.

[132] Niggli V. Signaling to migration in neutrophils: importance of localized pathways. Int J Biochem Cell Biol 2003; 35: 1619-38.

[133] Niggli V. Microtubule-disruption-induced and chemotactic-peptide-induced migration of human neutrophils: implications for differential sets of signaling pathways. J Cell Sci 2003; 116: 813-22.

[134] Penela P, Ribas C, Mayor F Jr. Mechanisms of regulation of the expression and function of G protein-coupled receptor kinases. Cell Signal 2003; 15: 973-81.

[135] Fan J, Malik AB. Toll-like receptor-4 (TLR4) signaling augments chemokine-induced neutrophil migration by modulating cell surface expression of chemokine receptors. Nat Med 2003; 9: 315-21.

[136] Arraes SM, Freitas MS, da Silva SV, *et al.* Impaired neutrophil chemotaxis in sepsis associates with GRK expression and inhibition of actin assembly and tyrosine phosphorylation. Blood 2006; 108: 2906-13.

[137] Hirsch E, Katanaev VL, Garlanda C, *et al.* Central role for G protein-coupled phosphoinositide 3-kinase gamma in inflammation. Science 2000; 287: 1049-53.

[138] Imose M, Nagaki M, Naiki T, *et al.* Inhibition of nuclear factor kappaB and phosphatidylinositol 3-kinase/Akt is essential for massive hepatocyte apoptosis induced by tumor necrosis factor alpha in mice. Liver Int 2003; 23: 386-96.

[139] Schabbauer G, Tencati M, Pedersen B, Pawlinski R, Mackman N. PI3K-Akt pathway suppresses coagulation and inflammation in endotoxemic mice. Arterioscler Thromb Vasc Biol 2004; 24: 1963-9.

[140] Yum HK, Arcaroli J, Kupfner J, *et al.* Involvement of phosphoinositide 3-kinases in neutrophil activation and the development of acute lung injury. J Immunol 2001; 167: 6601-8.

[141] Hoek JB, Pastorino JG. Cellular signaling mechanisms in alcohol-induced liver damage. Semin Liver Dis 2004; 24: 257-72.

[142] Alloatti G, Montrucchio G, Lembo G, Hirsch E. Phosphoinositide 3-kinase gamma: kinase-dependent and -independent activities in cardiovascular function and disease. Biochem Soc Trans 2004; 32: 383-6.

[143] Andrews S, Stephens LR, Hawkins PT. PI3K class IB pathway in neutrophils. Sci STKE. 2007; 2007(407):cm3.

[144] Martin EL, Souza DG, Fagundes CT, et al. PI3K{gamma} Kinase Activity Contributes to Sepsis and Organ Damage by Altering Neutrophil Recruitment. Am J Respir Crit Care Med 2010; [Epub ahead of print].

[145] Schmitz J, Owyang A, Oldham E, et al. IL-33, an interleukin-1-like cytokine that signals via the IL-1 receptor-related protein ST2 and induces T helper type 2-associated cytokines. Immunity 2005; 23: 479-90.

[146] Ali S, Huber M, Kollewe C, Bischoff SC, Falk W, Martin MU. IL-1 receptor accessory protein is essential for IL-33-induced activation of T lymphocytes and mast cells. Proc Natl Acad Sci USA 2007; 104: 18660-5.

[147] Chackerian AA, Oldham ER, Murphy EE, Schmitz J, Pflanz S, Kastelein RA. IL-1 receptor accessory protein and ST2 comprise the IL-33 receptor complex. J Immunol 2007; 179: 2551-5.

[148] Löhning M, Stroehmann A, Coyle AJ, et al. T1/ST2 is preferentially expressed on murine Th2 cells, independent of interleukin 4, interleukin 5, and interleukin 10, and important for Th2 effector function. Proc Natl Acad Sci U S A 1998; 95: 6930-5.

[149] Coyle AJ, Lloyd C, Tian J, et al. Crucial role of the interleukin 1 receptor family member T1/ST2 in T helper cell type 2-mediated lung mucosal immune responses. J Exp Med 1999; 190: 895-902.

[150] Brint EK, Xu D, Liu H, et al. ST2 is an inhibitor of interleukin 1 receptor and Toll-like receptor 4 signaling and maintains endotoxin tolerance. Nat Immunol 2004; 5: 373-9.

[151] Liew FY, Liu H, Xu D. A novel negative regulator for IL-1 receptor and Toll-like receptor 4. Immunol Lett 2005; 96: 27-31.

[152] Alves-Filho JC, Sônego F, Souto FO, et al. Interleukin-33 attenuates sepsis by enhancing neutrophil influx to the site of infection. Nat Med 2010; 16: 708-12.

[153] Moreno SE, Alves-Filho JC, Rios-Santos F, et al. Signaling via platelet-activating factor receptors accounts for the impairment of neutrophil migration in polymicrobial sepsis. J Immunol 2006; 177: 1264-71.

[154] Ishii S, Shimizu T. Platelet-activating factor (PAF) receptor and genetically engineered PAF receptor mutant mice. Prog Lipid Res 2000; 39: 41-82.

[155] Prescott SM, Zimmerman GA, Stafforini DM, McIntyre TM. Platelet-activating factor and related lipid mediators. Annu Rev Biochem 2000; 69: 419-45.

[156] Bulger EM, Arbabi S, Garcia I, Maier RV. The macrophage response to endotoxin requires platelet activating factor. Shock 2002; 17: 173-9.

[157] Stafforini DM, McIntyre TM, Zimmerman GA, Prescott SM. Platelet-activating factor acetylhydrolases. J Biol Chem 1997; 272: 17895-8.

[158] Karasawa K, Harada A, Satoh N, Inoue K, Setaka M. Plasma platelet activating factor-acetylhydrolase (PAF-AH). Prog Lipid Res 2003; 42: 93-114.

[159] Klein A, Talvani A, Silva PM, et al. Stem cell factor-induced leukotriene B4 production cooperates with eotaxin to mediate the recruitment of eosinophils during allergic pleurisy in mice. J Immunol 2001; 167: 524-31.

[160] Chou RC, Kim ND, Sadik CD, et al. Lipid-cytokine-chemokine cascade drives neutrophil recruitment in a murine model of inflammatory arthritis. Immunity 2010; 33: 266-78.

[161] Levy MM, Fink MP, Marshall JC, et al. 2001 SCCM/ESICM/ACCP/ATS/SIS International Sepsis Definitions Conference. Crit Care Med 2003; 31: 1250-6.

[162] Ognibene FP, Martin SE, Parker MM, et al. Adult respiratory distress syndrome in patients with severe neutropenia. N Engl J Med 1986; 315: 547-51.

[163] Miotla JM, Williams TJ, Hellewell PG, Jeffery PK. A role for the beta2 integrin CD11b in mediating experimental lung injury in mice. Am J Respir Cell Mol Biol 1996; 14: 363-73.

[164] Maunder RJ, Hackman RC, Riff E, Albert RK, Springmeyer SC. Occurrence of the adult respiratory distress syndrome in neutropenic patients. Am Rev Respir Dis 1986; 133: 313-6.

[165] van Eeden SF, Kitagawa Y, Klut ME, Lawrence E, Hogg JC. Polymorphonuclear leukocytes released from the bone marrow preferentially sequester in lung microvessels. Microcirculation 1997; 4: 369-80.

[166] Worthen GS, Schwab B 3rd, Elson EL, Downey GP. Mechanics of stimulated neutrophils: cell stiffening induces retention in capillaries. Science 1989; 245: 183-6.

[167] Worthen GS, Henson PM. Mechanisms of acute lung injury. Worthen GS, Henson PM. Clin Lab Med 1983; 3: 601-17.

[168] Bosken CH, Doerschuk CM, English D, Hogg JC. Neutrophil kinetics during active cigarette smoking in rabbits. J Appl Physiol 1991; 71: 630-7.

[169] Doerschuk CM. Mechanisms of leukocyte sequestration in inflamed lungs. Microcirculation 2001; 8: 71-88.

[170] Kang I, Wang Q, Eppell SJ, Marchant RE, Doerschuk CM. Effect of Neutrophil Adhesion on the Mechanical Properties of Lung Microvascular Endothelial Cells. Am J Respir Cell Mol Biol 2009; [Epub ahead of print].

[171] McDonald B, McAvoy EF, Lam F, *et al.* Interaction of CD44 and hyaluronan is the dominant mechanism for neutrophil sequestration in inflamed liver sinusoids. J Exp Med 2008; 205: 915-27.

[172] Clark SR, Ma AC, Tavener SA, *et al.* Platelet TLR4 activates neutrophil extracellular traps to ensnare bacteria in septic blood. Nat Med 2007; 13: 463-9.

[173] Cowburn AS, Condliffe AM, Farahi N, Summers C, Chilvers ER. Advances in neutrophil biology: clinical implications. Chest 2008; 134: 606-12.

[174] Astiz ME, DeGent GE, Lin RY, Rackow EC. Microvascular function and rheologic changes in hyperdynamic sepsis. Crit Care Med 1995; 23: 265-71.

[175] van der Poll T, Opal SM. Host-pathogen interactions in sepsis. Lancet Infect Dis 2008; 8: 32-43.

[176] Massberg S, Grahl L, von Bruehl ML, *et al.* Reciprocal coupling of coagulation and innate immunity via neutrophil serine proteases. Nat Med 2010; 16: 887-96.

CHAPTER 4

The Role of Neutrophils in *Chlamydia pneumoniae* Infection: First Line of Defense or the Gateway for Systemic Dissemination?

Ger van Zandbergen[1] and Jan Rupp[2,3,*]

[1]Institute for Medical Microbiology and Hygiene, University Clinic of Ulm; [2]Institute of Medical Microbiology and Hygiene, Germany and [3]Medical Clinic III, University Hospital Schleswig-Holstein/ Campus Lübeck, Germany

Abstract: The obligate intracellular bacterial pathogen *Chlamydia pneumoniae* (*Cpn*) is an established pathogen in acute lung infections. Recruitment of polymorphonuclear neutrophil granulocytes (PMN) to the lung is one of the first events upon acute infection. The functional role of PMN in *Cpn* pathogenicity and clearance is unclear. *In vitro* studies showed that *Cpn* stays alive after internalization by PMN in an opsonin-independent manner and are still able to multiply. While uninfected granulocytes become apoptotic, the lifespan of *Cpn* infected PMN is dramatically increased for more than 3 days. Ingestion of *Cpn* is accompanied by a complete re-programming of central PMN effector functions which are involved in cell survival, pathogen clearance and innate immunity. *In vivo* observations in rabbits suggest that PMN are centrally involved in the systemic dissemination of *Cpn* to the blood after acute lung infection. Furthermore, depletion of PMN in the lung seems to hamper chlamydial growth and progeny in the lung. In this review we will summarize studies on direct interactions of *Cpn* and PMN both *in vitro* and *in vivo*. Accumulating evidence suggest a central role of PMN in the systemic dissemination of *Cpn* infection.

INTRODUCTION

Since its first description in 1986, *Chlamydia pneumoniae* (*Cpn*) has emerged as an established cause of infections of the upper and lower respiratory tract [1]. Clinical appearance include cases of community acquired pneumonia, pharyngitis and sinusitis [2]. Since viable chlamydiae have been cultivated from atherosclerotic plaques and cerebrospinal fluid, *Cpn* has also been associated with several non-respiratory diseases such as coronary heart disease [3], multiple sclerosis [4], or Alzheimer's disease [5]. The mode of *Cpn* infection transmission from the lung, as the site of primary infection, to different organ tissues is still not completely understood. Although experimental intratracheal infection with *Cpn* results in a massive recruitment of polymorphonuclear neutrophil granulocytes (PMN), the role of these cells in the defense against *Cpn* is unclear. In this review we will summarize recent observations regarding direct interactions between *C. pneumoniae* and PMN *in vitro* and *in vivo*, and speculate on the function of PMN in *C. pneumoniae* infections.

UPTAKE, SURVIVAL AND APOPTOSIS REGULATION OF *CPN* IN PMN

As an obligate intracellular bacterium *Cpn* growth and progeny depends on the intracellular developmental phase, which lasts up to 72 hours. Preferred host cells of chlamydiae are epithelial cells, but infections of myeloid cells and even lymphocytes have been described [6]. *Cpn* infection of the lung was reported to activate airway epithelial cells and induce the release of IL-8 followed by a rapid transendothelial migration of PMN. Consequently, in the lung, PMN are among the first leukocytes to encounter *Cpn* [7-9]. PMN are inherently short-lived cells with a half-life of only about 6-10 hours in the circulation, after which they undergo spontaneous apoptosis [10]. However, in co-incubation experiments it was shown that PMN are able to internalize *Cpn* in an opsonin-independent manner and that the phagocytosed *Cpn* were not killed. Although at a low percentage, some of the ingested bacteria survived, multiplied and retained full virulence in PMN [11]. The finding that chlamydiae were able to replicate in PMN implicated that the life span of PMN must have been prolonged by the pathogen itself. Thus, co- incubation with *Cpn* resulted in a delay of neutrophil apoptosis for up to 3 days. Cellular apoptotic processes are well regulated and are characterized by cell shrinkage, chromatin condensation, internucleosomal DNA fragmentation, membrane blebbing and, finally, the decay into apoptotic bodies [12]. Although apoptosis is an intrinsic cell process, exogenous signals are strong mediators of apoptosis. For example, the life span of mature neutrophils can be extended *in vitro* by incubation with either proinflammatory cytokines including GM-CSF, G-CSF, IL-8, IL-1β or bacterial products such as lipopolysaccharide (LPS) [13-15]. The observed effect in *Cpn* infected PMN was

---

Address correspondence to Jan Rupp at: Medical Clinic III, University Hospital Schleswig-Holstein/ Campus Lübeck, Ratzeburger Allee 160, D-23562, Germany; E-mail: Jan.Rupp@uk-sh.de

mediated by both *Cpn* LPS and the autocrine IL-8 production of PMN [16]. Whereas *Cpn* LPS had the strongest anti-apoptotic effect up to 42 hours after *Cpn*- PMN co- incubation, increased release of IL-8 mediated the apoptosis inhibition at longer time intervals. The observed anti-apoptotic effects were associated with a markedly lower level of pro- caspase 3 processing and, consequently, a reduced caspase-3 activity in infected PMN [16]. Subsequently, extracellular phosphatidylserine (PS) expression as an early marker of the onset of apoptosis was delayed up to 42 hours p.i. Moreover, DNA degradation assessed by the TUNEL assay, as the final stage of apoptosis was delayed up to 42 hours p.i. [16]. Focussing on the mechanism of apoptosis delay in human neutrophils we found an increased stabilization in *Cpn* infected PMN of the anti-apoptotic Bcl-2 family member mcl-1 42 hours p.i. (Fig. **1**).

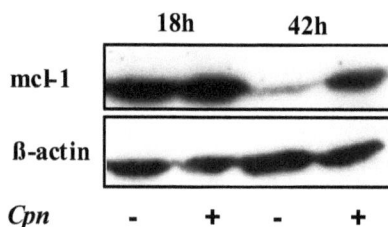

Figure 1: *Cpn* stabilizes mcl-1 in PMN. *Cpn* induced delay of apoptotic signaling in infected PMN is characterized by enhanced stabilization of mcl-1 (42h p.i), compared to non- infected control cells (representative experiment, n=3).

However, the functional role of mcl-1 stabilization in the mediation of apoptosis resistence in *Cpn* infected cells remains controversial. It seems to depend not only on the investigated host cells but also on the external stimulus which was used to induce cellular apoptosis [17,18].

Taken together, *Cpn* can extend the life span of neutrophil granulocytes making them suitable host cells for survival and multiplication within the first hours/days after infection, in contrast to other microbial pathogens that drive phagocytes into apoptosis in order to escape killing.

TRANSMISSION OF *CPN* INFECTION FROM PMN TO OTHER CELLS

It has been suggested that chlamydiae can benefit from a silent uptake resulting in increased survival and growth [19]. The most extensively studied example of a silent uptake into phagocytes is the clearance of apoptotic cells which is a well organized three step process [20]. First, apoptotic cells release "find-me" signals to recruit phagocytes to the site of apoptotic death [21]. Second, phagocytes recognize the presence of PS termed as "eat-me" signals on the membrane of apoptotic cells [20]. The final step is an active suppression of inflammation and immune response and can be termed as a "forget me" signal. This step is characterized by the release of the anti-inflammatory cytokine TGF-ß and down regulation of the pro-inflammatory cytokine TNF-α. Consequently, the clearance of apoptotic cells prevents immune responses against abundantly internalized and processed proteins of the apoptotic remains [22]. Chlamydiae apparently misuses this mechanism to be taken up from blood-derived macrophages (MF) inside apoptotic PMN [23]. First, the *Cpn* infection increased the capacity of PMN to release apoptotic "find me" signals attracting circulating MFs. *Cpn* hiding inside apoptotic PMN that expressed increased "eat me" signals on their surface are then taken up by phagocytic MFs. *Cpn* infection of MFs via apoptotic PMN finally induced the secretion of TGF-ß while the secretion of pro-inflammatory cytokines was hampered [23]. A response that could be named: "forget me" signal. It is postulated that the three step apoptotic transfer of *Cpn* allows the pathogen to be silently taken up in blood monocytes/macrophages that disseminate the pathogen throughout the organism.

TRANSFER OF *CPN* INFECTION TO MF BY APOPTOTIC PMN ALTER SUSCEPTIBILITY TO IFN-γ

Infection of myeloid cells with *Cpn* is a strong inducer of a pro-inflammatory immune response [24, 25]. However, freshly isolated monocytes resisted the development of infectious progeny, irrespective of whether tryptophan was added or the IFN-γ induced immune response was blocked by mAB [26]. Importantly, chlamydiae remained metabolically active and retained the capability to induce a positive lymphocyte proliferative response for up to 7 days [26, 27]. In contrast, high doses of IFN-γ clearly restricted the production of infectious progeny of *Cpn* in human monocyte-derived MF [28]. Thus, in activated cells, chlamydiae are either killed or a persistence-like state of infection develops. Intracellular viability and progeny of chlamydiae was recently linked to the JAK/STAT signaling pathway of infected host cells. It was found that chlamydial growth in epithelial cells nicely correlated with Stat-1 phosphorylation [29]. Moreover, *Cpn* infection *in vivo* revealed an infection dependent increase in Stat-1 phosphorylation in MF and dendritic cells [29, 30]. We could demonstrate increased activation of Stat-1 (Tyr701) in MF 90h p.i.. *Cpn* infection of MFs by the transfer of apoptotic PMN induced more Stat-1 phosphorylation when compared to direct infection of MF *Cpn* infection (Fig. **2**). On the other hand, masking PS with AnxA5 markedly reduced Stat-1 phosphorylation in MF infected with *Cpn* via PMN, suggesting a decreased chlamydial replication in MF after PS blocking on infected PMN (Fig. **2**).

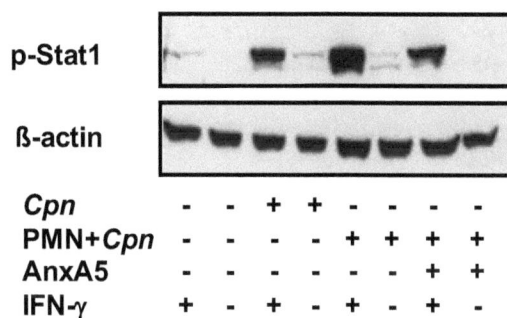

p-Stat1								
ß-actin								
Cpn	-	-	+	+	-	-	-	-
PMN+*Cpn*	-	-	-	-	+	+	+	+
AnxA5	-	-	-	-	-	-	+	+
IFN-γ	+	-	+	-	+	-	+	-

Figure 2: Increased phophorylation of Stat-1 by apoptotic transfer *Cpn* alone or *Cpn*-infected PMN (66 hours) with or without AnxA5 were co-incubated with autologous MF with 1 IFU or PMN. After 90 hours of culture MF were treated with IFN-γ (100U/ml) for 6 h or left in medium alone. MF lysates were analyzed by western blot for phosphorylated Stat-1 and ß-actin as a loading control (representative experiment, n=3).

HOST-DEFENSE STRATEGIES AND SYSTEMIC DISSEMINATION MEDIATED BY PMN

Activation of human airway epithelial cells and subsequent recruitment of PMN are the key steps in acute immune responses against respiratory pathogens in the lung. Thus, infection of primary human airway epithelial cells with *Cpn* not only resulted in a time- dependent induction of IL-8 and PGE2, but also increased the expression of the intercellular adhesion molecule-1 (ICAM-1) [31]. Subsequent transepithelial migration could be blocked by an anti-ICAM-1 mAB but not by mABs against IL-8 [31]. As chlamydial infections are also found in non-respiratory cells and organ tissues like peripheral blood monocytes (PBMC), the arterial vasculature or the brain, it is evident that the pathogen is systemically disseminated from the lung. Cell types involved in the dissemination are still insufficiently characterized. Some years ago, Gieffers *et al.* analyzed initial *Cpn* lung infection and subsequent systemic dissemination in a rabbit model of intratracheal *Cpn* infection [32]. Based on immunohistochemical analysis *Cpn* infection of the lung was divided into an early and late phase dominated by granulocytes or MF, respectively. Bronchiolar and alveolar epithelial cells, granulocytes, and MF were identified as primary target cells in acute *Cpn* lung infection [32]. During the later course of the infection, *Cpn* were detected inside MF systemically distributed in the peribronchial lymph nodes, spleen and the aortic vessel wall [32]. Rodriguez *et al.* could show that PMN that were recruited in the early phase of the *Cpn* lung infection in mice did not restrict chlamydial growth but rather improved replication of the pathogen [33]. Early immune responses triggered by *Cpn* partially depended on TLR2, but not on TLR4 [34]. A second mechanism by which PMN might be involved in the local spread of infectious chlamydiae has described recently. Using the guinea-pig conjunctival model of *Chlamydia caviae* Rank *et al.* could show that the adherence of infected epithelial cells with the basal lamina is disconnected as PMN infiltration intensifies in the diseased tissue [35]. As a result, PMN released infected superficial epithelia from the mucosa which in theory could move to new tissue sites [35].

CONCLUSIONS

Antibacterial effector functions of PMN have been extensively studied [36]. Differences in the effectiveness of these functions against extra- and intracellular bacteria became apparent recently. Thus, obligate intracellular bacteria like *Cpn* increase the life span of otherwise short-lived PMN to propagate. Intracellular survival of *Cpn* in PMN is characterized by increased expression of genes involved in pathogen metabolism and replication. Blood monocytes and MF have been shown to be centrally involved in systemic dissemination of *Cpn* from the lung to extrapulmonary organs. However, it is assumed that *Cpn* which develop a persistent-like state inside PBMC/MF, that is a least partially resistant to antibiotic treatment, will not survive over a long period of time [27, 37, 38]. Recent data now suggest that *Cpn* increases infectivity and bacterial load in PBMC/MF when the infection is transferred via apoptotic PMN [23]. Although experimental evidence was lacking, it has been suggested previously that chlamydiae might profit from hiding inside apoptotic cells [19]. First evidence supporting this hypothesis was reported from Ying *et al.* who could demonstrate that *Cpn* infection is transferred from UV-killed and PS-positive mouse embryonic fibroblast to mouse dendritic cells [39].

Regarding acute *Cpn* lung infections, it seems to be a footrace between direct clearance of *Cpn* by alveolar macrophages (AM) and the ingestion of *Cpn* by PMN that might increase chlamydial pathogenicity. Whether direct clearance of *Cpn* by MF results in complete eradication of the pathogen or promotes persistence of chlamydiae in the lung still has to be determined. Morphological analysis of *Cpn* inclusions in AM from *Cp*-DNA positive BAL-fluids indicate that direct and in-direct ingestion of chlamydiae might occur *in vivo*. Based on the fact that *C. pneumoniae* are not efficiently killed by PMN, novel strategies are warranted to treat systemic and persistent infections.

REFERENCES

[1]   Grayston JT, Kuo CC, Wang SP, Altman J. A new Chlamydia psittaci strain, TWAR, isolated in acute respiratory tract infections. N Engl J Med 1986; 315(3):161-8.

[2]   Kuo CC, Jackson LA, Campbell LA, Grayston JT. Chlamydia pneumoniae (TWAR). Clin Microbiol Rev 1995; 8(4):451-61.

[3]   Maass M, Bartels C, Engel PM, Mamat U, Sievers HH. Endovascular presence of viable Chlamydia pneumoniae is a common phenomenon in coronary artery disease. J Am Coll Cardiol 1998; 31(4):827-32.

[4]   Sriram S, Stratton CW, Yao S, *et al.* Chlamydia pneumoniae infection of the central nervous system in multiple sclerosis. Ann Neurol 1999; 46(1):6-14.

[5]   Balin BJ, Gerard HC, Arking EJ, *et al.* Identification and localization of Chlamydia pneumoniae in the Alzheimer's brain. Med Microbiol Immunol 1998; 187(1):23-42.

[6]   Kaul R, Uphoff J, Wiedeman J, Yadlapalli S, Wenman WM. Detection of Chlamydia pneumoniae DNA in CD3+ lymphocytes from healthy blood donors and patients with coronary artery disease. Circulation 2000; 102(19):2341-6.

[7]   Krull M, Klucken AC, Wuppermann FN, *et al.* Signal transduction pathways activated in endothelial cells following infection with Chlamydia pneumoniae. J Immunol 1999; 162(8):4834-41.

[8]   Molestina RE, Miller RD, Ramirez JA, Summersgill JT. Infection of human endothelial cells with Chlamydia pneumoniae stimulates transendothelial migration of neutrophils and monocytes. Infect Immun 1999; 67(3):1323-30.

[9]   Wyrick PB, Knight ST, Paul TR, Rank RG, Barbier CS. Persistent chlamydial envelope antigens in antibiotic-exposed infected cells trigger neutrophil chemotaxis. J Infect Dis 1999; 179(4):954-66.

[10]   Payne CM, Glasser L, Tischler ME, *et al.* Programmed cell death of the normal human neutrophil: an *in vitro* model of senescence. Microsc Res Tech 1994; 28(4):327-44.

[11]   Register KB, Morgan PA, Wyrick PB. Interaction between Chlamydia spp. and human polymorphonuclear leukocytes *in vitro*. Infect Immun 1986; 52(3):664-70.

[12]   Squier MK, Sehnert AJ, Cohen JJ. Apoptosis in leukocytes. J Leukoc Biol 199; 57(1):2-10.

[13]   Cox G, Gauldie J, Jordana M. Bronchial epithelial cell-derived cytokines (G-CSF and GM-CSF) promote the survival of peripheral blood neutrophils *in vitro*. Am J Respir Cell Mol Biol 1992; 7(5):507-13.

[14]   Kettritz R, Gaido ML, Haller H, Luft FC, Jennette CJ, Falk RJ. Interleukin-8 delays spontaneous and tumor necrosis factor-alpha-mediated apoptosis of human neutrophils. Kidney Int 1998; 53(1):84-91.

[15]   Colotta F, Re F, Polentarutti N, Sozzani S, Mantovani A. Modulation of granulocyte survival and programmed cell death by cytokines and bacterial products. Blood 1992; 80(8):2012-20.

[16]   van Zandbergen G, Gieffers J, Kothe H, *et al.* Chlamydia pneumoniae multiply in neutrophil granulocytes and delay their spontaneous apoptosis. J Immunol 2004; 172(3):1768-76.

[17]   Rajalingam K, Sharma M, Lohmann C, *et al.* Mcl-1 is a key regulator of apoptosis resistance in Chlamydia trachomatis-infected cells. PLoS One 2008; 3(9):e3102.

[18]   Ying S, Christian JG, Paschen SA, Hacker G. Chlamydia trachomatis can protect host cells against apoptosis in the absence of cellular Inhibitor of Apoptosis Proteins and Mcl-1. Microbes Infect 2008; 10(1):97-101.

[19]   Byrne GI, Ojcius DM. Chlamydia and apoptosis: life and death decisions of an intracellular pathogen. Nat Rev Microbiol 2004; 2(10):802-8.

[20]   Lauber K, Blumenthal SG, Waibel M, Wesselborg S. Clearance of apoptotic cells: getting rid of the corpses. Mol Cell 2004; 14(3):277-87.

[21]   Lauber K, Bohn E, Krober SM, *et al.* Apoptotic cells induce migration of phagocytes via caspase-3-mediated release of a lipid attraction signal. Cell 2003; 113(6):717-30.

[22]   Fadok VA, Bratton DL, Konowal A, Freed PW, Westcott JY, Henson PM. Macrophages that have ingested apoptotic cells *in vitro* inhibit proinflammatory cytokine production through autocrine/paracrine mechanisms involving TGF-beta, PGE2, and PAF. J Clin Invest 1998; 101(4):890-8.

[23]   Rupp J, Pfleiderer L, Jugert C, *et al.* Chlamydia pneumoniae hides inside apoptotic neutrophils to silently infect and propagate in macrophages. PLoS One 2009; 4(6):e6020.

[24]   Heinemann M, Susa M, Simnacher U, Marre R, Essig A. Growth of Chlamydia pneumoniae induces cytokine production and expression of CD14 in a human monocytic cell line. Infect Immun 1996; 64(11):4872-5.

[25]   Kaukoranta-Tolvanen SS, Teppo AM, Laitinen K, Saikku P, Linnavuori K, Leinonen M. Growth of Chlamydia pneumoniae in cultured human peripheral blood mononuclear cells and induction of a cytokine response. Microb Pathog 1996; 21(3):215-21.

[26]   Airenne S, Surcel HM, Alakarppa H, *et al.* Chlamydia pneumoniae infection in human monocytes. Infect Immun 1999; 67(3):1445-9.

[27]   Gieffers J, Fullgraf H, Jahn J, *et al.* Chlamydia pneumoniae infection in circulating human monocytes is refractory to antibiotic treatment. Circulation 2001; 103(3):351-6.

[28]   Airenne S, Surcel HM, Bloigu A, Laitinen K, Saikku P, Laurila A. The resistance of human monocyte-derived macrophages to Chlamydia pneumoniae infection is enhanced by interferon-gamma. APMIS 2000 Feb;108(2):139-44.

[29]   Lad SP, Fukuda EY, Li J, de la Maza LM, Li E. Up-regulation of the JAK/STAT1 signal pathway during Chlamydia trachomatis infection. J Immunol 2005 Jun 1;174(11):7186-93.

[30]   Yang T, Stark P, Janik K, Wigzell H, Rottenberg ME. SOCS-1 protects against Chlamydia pneumoniae-induced lethal inflammation but hampers effective bacterial clearance. J Immunol 2008; 180(6):4040-9.

[31]   Jahn HU, Krull M, Wuppermann FN, *et al.* Infection and activation of airway epithelial cells by Chlamydia pneumoniae. J Infect Dis 2000; 182(6):1678-87.

[32]   Gieffers J, van Zandbergen G., Rupp J, *et al.* Phagocytes transmit Chlamydia pneumoniae from the lungs to the vasculature. Eur Respir J 2004; 23(4):506-10.

[33]   Rodriguez N, Fend F, Jennen L, *et al.* Polymorphonuclear neutrophils improve replication of Chlamydia pneumoniae *in vivo* upon MyD88-dependent attraction. J Immunol 2005; 174(8):4836-44.

[34]   Rodriguez N, Wantia N, Fend F, Durr S, Wagner H, Miethke T. Differential involvement of TLR2 and TLR4 in host survival during pulmonary infection with Chlamydia pneumoniae. Eur J Immunol 2006; 36(5):1145-55.

[35]   Rank RG, Whittimore J, Bowlin AK, ssus-Babus S, Wyrick PB. Chlamydiae and polymorphonuclear leukocytes: unlikely allies in the spread of chlamydial infection. FEMS Immunol Med Microbiol 2008; 54(1):104-13.

[36]   Soehnlein O. Direct and alternative antimicrobial mechanisms of neutrophil-derived granule proteins. J Mol Med 2009; 87(12):1157-64.

[37]   Gaydos CA, Summersgill JT, Sahney NN, Ramirez JA, Quinn TC. Replication of Chlamydia pneumoniae *in vitro* in human macrophages, endothelial cells, and aortic artery smooth muscle cells. Infect Immun 1996; 64(5):1614-20.

[38]   Wolf K, Fischer E, Hackstadt T. Degradation of Chlamydia pneumoniae by peripheral blood monocytic cells. Infect Immun 2005; 73(8):4560-70.

[39]   Ying S, Fischer SF, Pettengill M, *et al.* Characterization of host cell death induced by Chlamydia trachomatis. Infect Immun 2006; 74(11):6057-66.

CHAPTER 5

Neutrophils in Mycobacterial Infections

Angelo Martino[1], Edgar Badell[2] and Nathalie Winter[3],*

[1]National Institute for Infectious Diseases-IRCCS, Lazzaro Spallanzani, Rome, Italy; [2]Institut Pasteur, Unité de Génétique Mycobactérienne, 25 rue du Dr Roux, Paris, France and [3]INRA, U1282, Infectiologie Animale & Santé Publique, Nouzilly, France

Abstract: *Mycobacterium tuberculosis* is a major human pathogen responsible for about two million deaths per year. The only available vaccine is the live attenuated strain *M. bovis* Bacille Calmette Guérin (BCG) that partially protects against pulmonary tuberculosis (TB). Mycobacteria are intracellular pathogens that are able to parasitize macrophages. The inflammatory process induced by mycobacterial infection also recruits neutrophils. Although neutrophils may directly kill some bacilli, this is not the major control they exert on mycobacterial infections. Neutrophils are able to shuttle BCG to the draining lymph node. They crosstalk with dendritic cells to increase BCG antigen presentation and modify cytokine expression profile. Neutrophils help in the early organization of mycobacterial granulomas that are key structures to contain bacilli. However, neutrophils are Janus-like cells that also have detrimental effects on *Mycobaterium tuberculosis* (Mtb) infection. Neutrophil accumulation in lungs correlates with Mtb high susceptibility in mice and with active pulmonary TB in humans. Mouse neutrophils secrete anti-inflammatory IL-10 upon mycobacterial stimulation that counters Mtb control. Recent discoveries have shown that Myeloid Derived Suppressor Cells - another granulocytic cell population close to neutrophils and exerting strong T cell suppression – are also recruited upon BCG vaccination in the mouse model which opens new perspectives on the key role played by granulocytes on the mycobacterial immune control.

INTRODUCTION

One third of the world population is infected with *Mycobacterium tuberculosis* (Mtb) and each year, approximately two million people die of this dreadful pathogen [1]. The only vaccine available, the live attenuated strain *M. bovis* Bacillus Calmette-Guérin (BCG) efficiently protects against severe disseminated tuberculosis (TB) in children but its efficacy against pulmonary TB in young adults is variable. Thus, despite widespread vaccination, BCG has a moderate impact on global TB.

TB is a chronic lung disease. In most cases primary infection is well controlled by the host. However, Mtb has developed a full range of mechanisms to escape the macrophage defences and is able to persist for years in latent forms. Upon immunosuppressive conditions - the most severe being HIV co infection –TB may reactivate and fully develop in a clinical disease and active transmission. We face a huge reservoir of Mtb latently infected people worldwide which represents a sword of Damocles.

Some cellular aspects of TB physiopathology have been well characterized both in patients and suitable animal models. Mtb mostly targets lung alveolar macrophages, even though other innate cells such as dendritic cells (DCs) and neutrophils can also be infected with Mtb. Rapidly after Mtb entry in the lung, infected macrophages are surrounded by lymphocytes to help them combat intracellular Mtb; this starts the granulomatous response. The most prevalent view is that early granulomas restrain mycobacterial infection and prevent bacilli dissemination throughout the body. Th1 cytokines, mostly IFN-γ and TNF-α, are key factor in granuloma formation and in macrophage activation. In the mouse model, high-resolution multiplex static imaging and intravital multiphoton microscopy of early granulomas show highly mobile T lymphocytes, recruited upon TNF-derived signals, which maintain the granuloma structure [2] and control infection. Upon maturation, granulomas eventually breakdown and release Mtb into the airways. TNF is also involved in progression to active disease as too much TNF causes tissue destruction, caseation and necrosis.

Tissue or lymph node resident DCs loaded with mycobacterial antigens play important role in the early granuloma formation through T-cell priming. Mycobacteria display multiple inflammatory signals that also recruit neutrophils whose role is still debated. Neutrophils are often considered as unsophisticated cells that arrive swiftly to the infection site, kill as many bacteria as they can and are quickly disposed of by surrounding macrophages to avoid

---

Address correspondence to Nathalie Winter at: INRA, U1282, Infectiologie Animale & Santé Publique, 37380, Nouzilly, France; E-mail: nathalie.winter@tours.inra.fr

Fabienne Tacchini-Cottier and Ger van Zandbergen (Eds)

tissue damage. Yet, neutrophils are much more subtle and in several infectious processes, they are legitimate partners of the immune response [3]. Recent findings on the multifaceted roles played by neutrophils during mycobacterial infections emphasize this view.

NEUTROPHILS AS DIRECT MYCOBACTERIAL KILLERS

Despite the clear role of neutrophils to combat extracellular infections, their role against intracellular pathogens is more controversial: this holds true for mycobacteria. The early host response to Mtb infection involves primarily resident alveolar macrophages and recruited neutrophils. However the killing activity of neutrophils against virulent Mtb strains measured *in vitro*, has been inconsistent [4-6]. In infected patients, as well as in animal models neutrophils are actively recruited upon infection. Despite inefficient direct killing, after apoptosis they could arm infected macrophages with the transfer of granules containing antimicrobial agents, such as defensins and cathelicidin LL-37 [7]. Thus, in TB contact patients, risk of infection is inversely correlated with peripheral blood neutrophil count [8]. Since neutrophil-derived cathelicidin LL-37 and lipocalin 2 restrict mycobacterial growth *in vitro* these data indicate an important role for neutrophils in innate control of TB infection. Nevertheless, the role of neutrophils in mycobacterial control has been inconsistently reproduced in mouse models. Mice efficiently control Mtb infection even in absence of neutrophils [9] even though reconstitution with neutrophils helps them better control *Mycobacterium avium*, another mycobacterial species of importance in immuno-compromised patients [10]. Interestingly, upon mycobacterial infection neutrophils release extracellular traps (NETs) (see Chapter xx) that could also play a role in mycobacterial control [11].

TRAVELING NEUTROPHILS

Naïve T cells meet their cognate antigen in peripheral lymphoid organs, proliferate and travel back to the infected site to locally orchestrate the control of intracellular pathogens. The antigenic cargo has to travel from the entry point to the lymphoid organ to be presented to T cells by Antigen Presenting Cells (APCs). For a long time, DCs, the most professional APC, have been considered the unique travelling cells that are able to pick up the antigen in the tissue and transfer it to the draining lymph node. This view was challenged by a number of studies including our pioneering work on early immune events following BCG vaccination. We injected fluorescent reporter BCG strains in the mouse ear as a surrogate model for intradermal vaccination in human skin. Our hypothesis was that resident skin DCs would be the main cells involved in BCG capture and transfer to the draining lymph node. To our surprise, we observed that neutrophils were the main primary BCG-host cells in skin and lymph node. Moreover, infected neutrophils transporting BCG to the draining lymph node were tracked in lymphatic vessels demonstrating that the infected neutrophils recruited to skin upon inflammation were able to migrate to the lymph node [12]. This established that neutrophil fate is not only to die in the tissue. Traveling neutrophils are not restricted to BCG vaccination: they were observed in mice injected with the parasite *Toxoplasma gondii* [13], the nematode *Nippostrongylus brasiliensis* [14] or with purified protein ovalbumin [15]. Furthermore, they are not restricted to mice as sheep administered with *Salmonella abortusovis* in the oral mucosa exhibited infected neutrophils migrating in the afferent lymph [16]. Thus the paradigm has been defined that under some circumstances, neutrophils are able to carry antigens and/or pathogens to the draining lymph node where they meet with T cells. Indeed, in the lymph node draining BCG vaccination site, we observed neutrophils in close contact with DCs and T cells [12]. Notably, neutrophils efficiently cross-present antigens to naïve CD8 T cells [17, 18]. Neutrophils also acquire some features of professional APCs in certain conditions or can cooperate with DCs to enhance their antigen presentation capacities (see below).

THE BRIGHT SIDE OF NEUTROPHILS

Neutrophils are Essential Players in the Protective Immune Response against Mycobacteria

Activated neutrophils express a variety of cytokines and chemokines that orchestrate the immune response by modulating T cell polarisation and attracting cells to the site of infection. Neutrophils are primary cells recruited upon infection with Mtb in the lung [19] or vaccination with BCG [12] and efficiently engulf bacilli. Even though the neutrophils'role in direct mycobacterial killing is questionable, they are instrumental in early Th1 cell polarisation leading to macrophage activation because they secrete large amounts of IL-12 [10, 20]. Neutrophils are also apposed to DCs both in tissues and in lymph node [12] and thus ideally placed to crosstalk. We analyzed cell cooperation taking place between neutrophils and DCs in response to BCG infection both in human and mouse systems [21]. Upon physical contact, BCG-infected neutrophils deliver signals to DCs that accommodate their maturation and induce secretion of Tcell-activating cytokines. Moreover, T cell proliferation and IFN-γ secretion in response to DCs in contact with BCG-infected neutrophils are increased in comparison to the T cell response raised to directly infected DCs [21]. Therefore it is possible that a "ménage-à-trois" between neutrophils, acquiring BCG in skin and migrating to the draining lymph node where they encounter DCs and naïve T cells, promotes activation of the primary T cell response.

Neutrophils rapidly enter in apoptosis independently of their infection status. Whereas non-infected apoptotic neutrophils dampen DC activation, Mtb-infected neutrophils that enter in apoptosis, deliver maturation and activation signals to DCs [22] suggesting again a helper role for neutrophil to initiate the T cell response. Moreover, in the case of prolonged contact between T cells and neutrophils, such as in tuberculous pleuritis, neutrophils resisting apoptosis upregulate the expression of cell surface molecules involved in T cell activation such as CD83, CD86 and MHC-II present on DCs [23] indicating that neutrophils might directly present mycobacterial antigens to CD4 T cells. Therefore, despite a controversial direct role in Mtb control, early recruited neutrophils are involved in tailoring the immune response to Mtb at least through cooperation with other innate cells.

Neutrophils, IL-17A and Granuloma Formation

Locally formed granulomas are essential to control mycobacterial infection and dissemination through the body [24]. TNF is one key soluble factor involved in granuloma formation and control in animal models [25]. Humans under anti-TNF therapy present an increased risk to develop TB [26]. Regarding cells contributing to granuloma formation, several reports indicate an important role for early recruited neutrophils that contribute TNF production in mice [10, 20, 21, 27] and in guinea pigs, an animal model that is highly sensitive to Mtb [28]. Neutrophils are involved in granuloma formation by other mechanisms too. In mice, antibody-mediated neutrophil depletion performed at time of aerosol infection with virulent Mtb, exerts a strong negative effect on granuloma formation observed one month later. This early regulatory effect depends on chemokines, in particular MIG (CXCL9), signaling through CXCR3 expressed by CD4 Th1 lymphocytes [29].

IL-17A is a key factor in granulopoiesis and neutrophil recruitment [30]. Although Th17-derived IL-17A does not directly activate human neutrophils due to their defective IL-17RC receptor, Th17 cells can produce CXCL-8, a potent chemoattractant for neutrophils [31]. In BCG-vaccinated mice, Th17-derived IL-17A is an important regulator of protective Th1-cell recruitment to the lung following Mtb infection [32]. IL-17A is also produced during the innate phase of the response to infection, mainly by γδ T cells through direct recognition of pathogen-derived Pattern-Associated Molecular Patterns by Toll-Like receptors [33, 34]. Accordingly upon intranasal infection with BCG, γδ T cells are the primary IL-17A producers in the lung. In IL-17A$^{-/-}$ BCG-infected mice, the granuloma formation is highly compromised [35]. Granuloma maturation is also impaired in absence of IL-17A after Mtb infection in lungs which compromises bacilli growth restriction [36]. Similarly, mice genetically deficient for γδ T cells infected with *M. avium* [37, 38] do not develop protective granulomas. Neutrophils recruited via IL-17A produced by γδ T cells could thus represent an important regulatory component of early mycobacterial granuloma formation in lung upon Mtb infection. Interestingly, IL-17A is produced by neutrophils themselves in the context of different inflammatory disorders [39, 40]. Therefore, in animal models neutrophils appear to be the key cells in early protective granuloma formation against mycobacterial infection.

THE DARK SIDE OF NEUTROPHILS

Neutrophils are chronically recruited to lungs after Mtb infection. In the mouse model, during the first two weeks following Mtb aerogenic infection, neutrophils and macrophages are the predominant cell types in lungs. They sharply decline at 4 weeks post-infection and rise again after 12 weeks [19]. Thus early and late neutrophils might play distinct roles. Susceptibility to Mtb infection varies among different mice strains : I/StYCit, DBA/2 and CBA/J are highly susceptible to Mtb infection whereas C57/Bl6 and BALB/c resist better. In I/StYCit mice, an increased influx and a longer survival of neutrophils in infected lungs is correlated to increased pathology [41]. Gene expression analysis performed in Mtb susceptible and resistant mice reveals a bias towards the increased expression of IL-17R or sfpi involved in granulopoiesis and LIX (CXCL5) involved in granulocyte recruitment in susceptible mice [42]. Moreover when granulocytes are depleted, by injection of an antibody targeting the granulocyte-expressed molecule Gr1, Mtb susceptible DBA/2 mice survive longer to infection [42]. Repeated BCG vaccination of Mtb infected C57/Bl6 mice exacerbates IL-17A and IL-23 response in lungs. Granulocytes, most probably neutrophils, accumulate in lesions in response to IL-17A/IL-23 and lungs become highly necrotic [43]. Therefore, sustained neutrophil influx related to pathological IL-17A response, plays detrimental role in chronic TB. All these studies indicate that Mtb-induced destructive lung parenchyma inflammation correlates with unrestrained neutrophils exacerbating tissue damage. However, a recent study from Zhang *et al.* challenges this view. Indeed, after triggering with BCG, neutrophils secrete high amounts of anti-inflammatory IL-10, in contrast to monocytes that secrete pro-inflammatory cytokines. Mycobacterial derived carbohydrates trigger Syk kinase downstream from Dectins and MyD88 downstream from TLR2, which induce high amounts of IL-10 production by highly purified mouse neutrophils. This anti-inflammatory pathway down modulates BCG-induced lung inflammation in the acute phase and helps Mtb to persist in chronically infected mice [44]. Therefore according to these recent data, neutrophils are detrimental to Mtb control yet via anti-inflammatory mechanisms. Whether, IL-10 is also produced by human neutrophils in the context of Mtb infection and helps bacilli establishment is an interesting view that deserves investigation.

In TB-infected humans the neutrophil-attracting chemokine CXCL-8 is massively produced in lungs. IL-17A and IL-22 producing CD4+ T cells are detected in people exposed to Mtb which could also contribute to neutrophil recruitment. Neutrophils are indeed the predominant cells in airways from active pulmonary TB patients which engulf bacilli. Yet, they are unable to control Mtb replication. Interestingly, Eum *et al.* reported that intracellular Mtb replicate rapidly in patient neutrophils. Hence neutrophils could represent supportive cells for bacilli that promote active transmission [45].

Taken together these observations highlight the Janus-like nature of the neutrophilic response to mycobacterial infection. TB control requires the right cytokine balance and also a tightly controlled cell influx. The local cytokine environment probably plays a crucial role in neutrophil effector capacity in a similar way as has been described for macrophages that can be deactivated, classically or alternatively activated with different outcomes of intracellular infection control. Interestingly, in lung cancer two different neutrophil populations are described in tumors; "N1" neutrophils that inhibit or "N2" neutrophils that promote cancer development [46]. Whether similar neutrophil populations also occur in TB at different stages is unknown. However, neutrophils are definitely important regulators of both TB immune response and physiopathology.

NEUTROPHILS AND MORE …

Even though neutrophils egress from the bone marrow as mature and fully active cells, they keep some plasticity and display different phenotypes and functions depending on the infectious agent and host susceptibility to infection [47]. Neutrophils belong to a large family of myeloid cells termed "granulocytes". They are close relatives to monocytes/macrophages, a key cell in the control of mycobacterial infection. The most widely used cell surface marker to define mouse "neutrophils" by flow cytometry is by far Gr-1, corresponding to two glycosylphosphatidylinositol-anchored proteins : Ly-6C and Ly-6G. However, whereas Ly-6G expression is restricted to genuine neutrophils [48], Ly-6C is broadly expressed in additional immune cells, including T cells, DCs and monocytes. Therefore many studies based on the antibody RB6-8C5 binding to Gr1 claiming roles for neutrophils should be interpreted with caution (see chapter by Charmoy *et al.*). In cancer a heterogeneous set of immunosuppressive cells, highly resembling neutrophils and operationally defined as myeloid-derived suppressor cells (MDSCs) are recruited to the tumor site and lymphoid organs. Similar cells are also present during pathological inflammation such as sepsis [49]. MDSCs strongly suppress T cell proliferation via L-arginine dependent mechanisms such as nitric oxide, produced by the inducible Nitric Oxide Synthase (iNOS). Both neutrophils and MDSCs share Gr1 and CD11b cell surface expression. We have recently described that early after BCG skin inoculation in the mouse, the granulocytic infiltrate is composed of *bona fide* neutrophils and innate MDSCs (inMDSCs) [27]. Upon neutrophil-specific depletion, MDSC influx is widely increased suggesting a neutrophil-inMDSCs balanced recruitment in response to BCG injection. inMDSC require MyD88 signalling to invade skin whereas neutrophil influx is MyD88-independent. inMDSCs are only able to produce iNOS through IL-1 receptor signalling. Despite elevated NO production, inMDSCs are unable to restrict BCG multiplication. In agreement with MDSC function observed in cancer or sepsis, inMDSCs strongly suppress T cells via NO-dependent mechanisms, which dampens *in vivo* BCG-specific T-cell priming. Thus, BCG vaccination induces a balanced neutrophil-inMDSC recruitment to skin and draining lymph node. We suggest that inMDSCs serve two functions. First, since they are unable to destroy mycobacteria but strongly block T-cell priming, they might represent a niche for BCG to establish in the host. Second, inMDSCs might restrain exuberant T cell proliferation and cytokine production to avoid tissue inflammation. Whether similar cells are also present during Mtb infection in the mouse model and in humans is not known at present. If they were, one could speculate that inMDSC could counterbalance neutrophils during the different phases of Mtb infection especially for the early formation and late breakdown of the granuloma.

CONCLUDING REMARKS

Clinical studies and experimental infections have shown that acute pulmonary TB is accompanied by an influx of neutrophils. However the published literature leaves us with a contradictory picture of the neutrophil's role in the host defence against mycobacterial infections. This is in relation to the Janus-like profile of neutrophils that on the one hand are the most rapid and effective cells to reach a tissue upon insult to combat an infection but on the other hand must be tightly controlled to avoid tissue damage. Recent literature highlights that neutrophils must be considered for their potent immunoregulatory role during mycobacterial infection. Immunoregulation again displays a double-faced profile depending on models, mycobacterial strains, kinetics of infection, etc. Neutrophils are now being classified in distinct subsets that, similarly to DCs or macrophages, probably display distinct immunoregulatory roles during mycobacterial infections. Moreover, the recruitment to the infection site of neutrophil-"sister" cells such as the recently described MDSCs, have probably been overlooked in previous studies due to the lack of specific markers. Knockout mice deficient for these various cell types and subsets will probably help to clarify the picture in the near future.

Extrapolation from *in vivo* observations in mice to clinical situation in humans remains challenging. New non-invasive techniques are required to observe neutrophils *in situ* in humans. New diagnostic tools allowing Mtb infection detection at very early times are also needed. Probably a more realistic view, if we want to get a clearer picture of the role of neutrophils during the whole course of Mtb infection, is to develop innovative preclinical animal models other than mice, and developing TB with clinical features closer to that observed in humans.

In conclusion, the role of neutrophils during mycobacterial infections still puzzles us. What is now clear is the plasticity and regulatory functions of neutrophils in immune reactions that must be taken in to account to clarify the complex picture of interactions Mtb plays with its host.

ACKNOWLEDGEMENTS

This work was supported by European Union Contract LSHP-CT-2003-503240 MUVAPRED and by the French Agence Nationale de la Recherche Contract ANR-08-MIEN-001.

REFERENCES

[1]   Dye C. Global epidemiology of tuberculosis. Lancet 2006; 367: 938-40.
[2]   Egen JG, Rothfuchs AG, Feng CG, Winter N, Sher A, Germain RN. Macrophage and T cell dynamics during the development and disintegration of mycobacterial granulomas. Immunity 2008; 28(2):271-84
[3]   Nathan C. Neutrophils and immunity: challenges and opportunities. Nat Rev Immunol 2006; 6: 173-82.
[4]   Brown AE, Holzer TJ, Andersen BR. Capacity of human neutrophils to kill Mycobacterium tuberculosis. J Infect Dis 1987; 156(6):985-9.
[5]   Denis M. Human neutrophils, activated with cytokines or not, do not kill virulent Mycobacterium tuberculosis. J Infect Dis 1991; 163: 919-20.
[6]   Jones GS, Amirault HJ, Andersen BR. Killing of Mycobacterium tuberculosis by neutrophils: a nonoxidative process. J Infect Dis 1990; 162(3): 700-4.
[7]   Tan BH, Meinken C, Bastian M, *et al.* Macrophages acquire neutrophil granules for antimicrobial activity against intracellular pathogens. J Immunol 2006; 177(3): 1864-71.
[8]   Martineau AR, Newton SM, Wilkinson KA, *et al.* Neutrophil-mediated innate immune resistance to mycobacteria. J Clin Invest 2007; 117(7): 1988-94.

[9]   Seiler P, Aichele P, Raupach B, Odermatt B, Steinhoff U, Kaufmann SH. Rapid neutrophil response controls fast-replicating intracellular bacteria but no slow-replicating Mycobacterium tuberculosis. J Infec Dis 2000; 181(2): 671-80.

[10]   Pedrosa J, Saunders BM, Appelberg R, Orme IM, Silva MT, Cooper AM. Neutrophils play a protective nonphagocytic role in systemic Mycobacterium tuberculosis infection of mice. Infect Immun 2000; 68(2): 577-83.

[11]   Ramos-Kichik V, Mondragón-Flores R, Mondragón-Castelán M, et al. Neutrophil extracellular traps are induced by Mycobacterium tuberculosis. Tuberculosis 2009; 89(1): 29-37.

[12]   Abadie V, Badell E, Douillard P, et al. Neutrophils rapidly migrate via lymphatics after Mycobacterium bovis BCG intradermal vaccination and shuttle live bacilli to the draining lymph nodes. Blood 2005; 106(5): 1843-50.

[13]   Chtanova T, Schaeffer M, Han SJ, et al. Dynamics of neutrophil migration in lymph nodes during infection. Immunity 2008; 29(3): 487-96.

[14]   Pesce JT, Liu Z, Hamed H, et al. Neutrophils clear bacteria associated with parasitic nematodes augmenting the development of an effective Th2-type response. J Immunol 2008; 180(1): 464-74.

[15]   Maletto BA, Ropolo AS, Alignani DO, et al. Presence of neutrophil-bearing antigen in lymphoid organs of immune mice. Blood 2006; 108(9): 3094-102.

[16]   Bonneau M, Epardaud M, Payot F, et al. Migratory monocytes and granulocytes are major lymphatic carriers of Salmonella from tissue to draining lymph node. J Leukoc Biol 2006; 79(2): 268-76.

[17]   Beauvillain C, Delneste Y, Scotet M. et al. Neutrophils efficiently cross-prime naive T cells in vivo. Blood 2007; 110(8): 2965-73.

[18]   Tvinnereim AR, Hamilton SE, Harty JT. Neutrophil involvement in cross-priming CD8+ T cell responses to bacterial antigens. J Immunol 2004; 173(3): 1994-2002.

[19]   Tsai MC, Chakravarty S, Zhu G, et al. Characterization of the tuberculous granuloma in murine and human lungs: cellular composition and relative tissue oxygen tension. Cell Microbiol 2006; 8(2): 218-32.

[20]   Petrofsky M, Bermudez LE. Neutrophils from Mycobacterium avium-infected mice produce TNF-α, IL-12, and IL-1β and have a putative role in early host response. Clin Immunol 1999; 91(3): 354-8.

[21]   Morel C, Badell E, Abadie V, et al. Mycobacterium bovis BCG-infected neutrophils and dendritic cells cooperate to induce specific T-cell responses in humans and mice. Eur J Immunol 2008; 38(2): 437-47.

[22]   Alemán M, de la Barrera S, Schierloh P, et al. Spontaneous or Mycobacterium tuberculosis-induced apoptotic neutrophils exert opposite effects on the dendritic cell-mediated immune response. Eur J Immunol 2007; 37(6): 1524-37.

[23]   Aleman M, de la Barrera SS, Schierloh PL, et al. In tuberculous pleural effusions, activated neutrophils undergo apoptosis and acquire a dendritic cell-like phenotype. J Infect Dis 2005; 192(3): 399-409.

[24]   Russell DG, Cardona PJ, Kim MJ, Allain S, Altare F. Foamy macrophages and the progression of the human tuberculous granuloma. Nat Immunol 2009; 10(9): 943-8.

[25]   Flynn JL, Goldstein MM, Chan J, et al. Tumor necrosis factor-alpha is required in the protective immune response against mycobacterium tuberculosis in mice. Immunity 1995; 2(6): 561-72.

[26]   Ehlers S, Why does tumor necrosis factor targeted therapy reactivate tuberculosis? J Rheumatol 2005; 32(74): 35-39.

[27]   Martino A, Badell E, Abadie V, et al. Mycobacterium bovis Bacillus Calmette-Guerin vaccination mobilizes innate Myeloid-Derived Suppressor Cells restraining in vivo T cell priming via IL-1R-dependent nitric oxide production. J Immunol 2010; 184(4): 2038-47.

[28]   Sawant KV, McMurray DN. Guinea pig neutrophils infected with Mycobacterium tuberculosis produce cytokines which activate alveolar macrophages in noncontact cultures. Infect Immun 2007; 75(4): 1870-7.

[29]   Seiler P, Aichele P, Bandermann S, et al. Early granuloma formation after aerosol Mycobacterium tuberculosis infection is regulated by neutrophils via CXCR3-signaling chemokines. Eur J Immunol 2003; 33(10): 2676-86.

[30]   Stark MA, Huo Y, Burcin TL, Morris MA, Olson TS, Ley K. Phagocytosis of apoptotic neutrophils regulates granulopoiesis via IL-23 and IL-17. Immunity 2005; 22(3): 285-94.

[31]   Pelletier M, Maggi L, Micheletti A, et al. Evidence for a cross-talk between human neutrophils and Th17 cells. Blood 2010; 115(2): 335-43.

[32]   Khader SA, Bell GK, Pearl JE, et al. IL-23 and IL-17 in the establishment of protective pulmonary CD4+ T cell responses after vaccination and during Mycobacterium tuberculosis challenge. Nat Immunol 2007; 8(4): 69-377.

[33]   Martin B, Hirota K, Cua DJ, Stockinger B, Veldhoen M. Interleukin-17-producing gamma-delta T cells selectively expand in response to pathogen products and environmental signals. Immunity 2009; 31(2): 321-30.

[34]   Sutton CE, Lalor SJ, Sweeney CM, Brereton CF, Lavelle EC, Mills KH. Interleukin-1 and IL-23 induce innate IL-17 production from gamma-delta T cells, amplifying Th17 responses and autoimmunity. Immunity 2009; 31(2): 331-41.

[35]   Umemura M, Yahagi A, Hamada S, et al. IL-17-mediated regulation of innate and acquired immune response against pulmonary Mycobacterium bovis Bacille Calmette-Guerin infection. J Immunol 2007; 178(6): 3786-96.

[36] Okamoto Yoshida Y, Umemura M, Yahagi A, *et al.* Essential role of IL-17A in the formation of a mycobacterial infection-induced granuloma in the lung. J Immunol 2010; 184(8): 4414-22.

[37] Saunders BM, Frank AA, Cooper AM, Orme IM. Role of gamma delta T cells in immunopathology of pulmonary Mycobacterium avium infection in mice. Infect Immun 1998; 66(11): 5508-14.

[38] Tanaka S, Itohara S, Sato M, Taniguchi T, Yokomizo Y. Reduced formation of granulomata in gamma delta T cell knockout BALB/c mice inoculated with Mycobacterium avium subsp. paratuberculosis. Vet Pathol 2000; 37(5): 415-21.

[39] Ferretti S, Bonneau O, Dubois GR, Jones CE, Trifilieff A, *et al.* IL-17, produced by lymphocytes and neutrophils, is necessary for lipopolysaccharide-induced airway neutrophilia: IL-15 as a possible trigger. J Immunol 2003; 170(4): 2106-12.

[40] Li L, Huang L, Vergis AL, *et al.* IL-17 produced by neutrophils regulates IFN-g-mediated neutrophil migration in mouse kidney ischemia-reperfusion injury. J Clin Invest 2009; 120(1): 331-42.

[41] Eruslanov EB, Lyadova IV, Kondratieva TK, *et al.* Neutrophil responses to Mycobacterium tuberculosis infection in genetically susceptible and resistant mice. Infect Immun 2005; 73(3): 1744-53.

[42] Keller C, Hoffmann R, Lang R, Brandau S, Hermann C, Ehlers S. Genetically determined susceptibility to tuberculosis in mice causally involves accelerated and enhanced recruitment of granulocytes. Infect Immun 2006; 74(7): 4295-309.

[43] Cruz A, Fraga AG, Fountain JJ, *et al.* Pathological role of interleukin 17 in mice subjected to repeated BCG vaccination after infection with Mycobacterium tuberculosis. J Exp Med 2010; 207(8): 1609-16.

[44] Zhang X, Majlessi L, Deriaud E, Leclerc C, Lo-Man R. Coactivation of Syk kinase and MyD88 adaptor protein pathways by bacteria promotes regulatory properties of neutrophils. Immunity 2009; 31(5): 761-71.

[45] Eum SY, Kong JH, Hong MS, *et al.* Neutrophils are the predominant infected phagocytic cells in the airways of patients with active pulmonary. TB Chest 2009; 137(1): 122-8.

[46] Fridlender ZG, Sun J, Kim S, *et al.* Polarization of tumor-associated neutrophil phenotype by TGF-beta: "N1" versus "N2" TAN. Cancer Cell 2009; 16(3): 183-94.

[47] Tsuda Y, Takahashi H, Kobayashi M, Hanafusa T, Herndon DN, Suzuki F. Three different neutrophil subsets exhibited in mice with different susceptibilities to infection by methicillin-resistant Staphylococcus aureus. Immunity 2004; 21(2): 215-26.

[48] Fleming TJ, Fleming ML, Malek TR, Selective expression of Ly-6G on myeloid lineage cells in mouse bone marrow. RB6-8C5 mAb to granulocyte-differenciation antigen (Gr-1) detects members of the Ly-6 family. J Immunol 1993; 151(5): 2399-408

[49] Gabrilovich DI, Nagaraj S, Myeloid-derived suppressor cells as regulators of the immune system. Nat Rev Immunol 2009; 9: 162-74.

CHAPTER 6

Role of Neutrophils in the Early Shaping of the *Leishmania major* Specific Immune Response in Experimental Murine Cutaneous Leishmaniasis

Mélanie Charmoy[1], Geneviève Milon[2] and Fabienne Tacchini-Cottier[1,*]

[1]*WHO Immunology Research and Training Center, Department of Biochemistry, University of Lausanne, Epalinges, Switzerland and* [2]*Institut Pasteur, Département de Parasitologie et Mycologie, Unité d'Immunophysiologie et Parasitisme Intracellulaire, Paris, France*

Abstract: The development of a protective immune response to microorganisms involves complex interactions between the host and the pathogen. The murine model of infection with *Leishmania major* (*L. major*) allows the study of the factors leading to the development of a protective immune response. Following infection with the protozoan parasite *L. major*, most strains of mice heal their lesions, while a few fail to control infection, both processes linked to the development of specific T helper subsets. The early events occurring during the first days following parasite inoculation are thought to be critical in the development of the *Leishmania*-specific immune response. Neutrophils are the first cells arriving massively to the site of infection, and recent evidence points to their role as organizers of the immune response, yet their specific role in this process remains elusive. Through interactions with cells present at the parasite inoculation site, and possibly within the draining lymph nodes, neutrophils could have an impact not only on the recruitment of inflammatory cells but also on the activation of local as well as newly migrated cells that will be crucial in shaping the *Leishmania*-specific immune response.

INTRODUCTION

Biology of *Leishmania* Infection

Infection with parasites of *Leishmania* species result in a spectrum of local or systemic pathogenic processes in humans and mammals. Overall, leishmaniasis afflicts around 12 million individuals in 88 countries worldwide (for recent reviews see [1-6]). Unveiling the determinants of the pathogenic processes that account for the spectrum of human leishmaniasis remains an important research objective. The perpetuation of *Leishmania* relies on two populations of organism including pool blood-feeding sand flies and mammal hosts. Mammals act as a source of blood for the female sand flies needed to produce their progeny. The development of *Leishmania* in the sand fly is initiated when a female has taken a blood meal from a mammal displaying, in the dermis, mononuclear leukocytic phagocytes and/or fibroblasts hosting the amastigote stage of the parasite. Once the blood meal containing intracellular *Leishmania* reaches the posterior midgut of the sand fly, *Leishmania* amastigotes exit the mammalian cells and differentiate into procyclic promastigotes with very short flagella. The parasite matures through several developmental stages within the sand fly digestive tract, as the promastigotes migrate from the posterior midgut to the foregut [7-12]. Thus a female sand fly harbors infectious extracellular flagellated *Leishmania* promastigotes in the foregut lumen and the most anterior part of their midgut lumen. When taking its blood meal, it deposits the invasive promastigotes within the mammal dermis. These metacyclic promastigotes are inoculated either with saliva or with saliva and a proteophosphoglycan (PPG)-rich gel secreted by non metacyclic promastigotes. The saliva delivery reflects that the *Leishmania*-hosting sand fly was only able to probe the skin, depositing a low number of motile metacyclic promastigotes. In contrast, inoculation with saliva and PPG-rich gel indicates that the sand fly was able to take its blood meal and regurgitate metacyclic promastigotes embedded in this gel. Rodent models act as hosts of at least the skin-tropic *Leishmania* species. Thus we set up experimental conditions in rodents to explore 1) the determinants of the transient or nonhealing skin lesion that can develop at the site of *Leishmania* inoculation 2) and the effect of *Leishmania* inoculation within the skin and the skin-draining lymph nodes of these infected mice. One of our objectives is to determine the vector, parasite and host factors that result in either clinically detectable transient tissue damage followed by repair, a process associated with *L. major* persistence; or asymptomatic stable and long term parasitism where the infected mammal host serves as a reservoir for the sand fly-invasive amastigote population.

In this chapter, we describe neutrophil biology in the bone marrow at steady state, and during the inflammatory response. Next, we compare the efficacy of several neutrophil-depleting monoclonal antibodies currently available,

Address correspondence to Fabienne Tacchini-Cottier at: WHO Immunology Research and Training Center, Department of Biochemistry, University of Lausanne, Boveresses 155, 1066 Epalinges, Switzerland; E-mail: fabienne.tacchini-cottier@unil.ch

as they are important tools to study the role of neutrophils in several models of infection. We then summarize data revealing how interactions between neutrophils and non neutrophil leukocyte subsets contribute to the early phase of *L. major* establishment, and influence the subsequent phases of the infection, including the immune response.

THE MOUSE BONE MARROW IN STEADY STATE: A SITE OF NEUTROPHIL GRANULOCYTE PRODUCTION, STORAGE, EGRESS AND CLEARANCE

In adult mammals, the bone marrow (BM) is the primary site for hematopoiesis [13, 14]. In the adult mouse, hematopoiesis gives rise to long-term reconstituting Hemopoietic Stem Cells (HSCs) that, in turn, generate short-term repopulating HSCs. From these stem cells, a number of more restricted progenitors (Hematopoietic Stem and Progenitor Cells (HSPCs)) emerge that give rise to all differentiated blood cells in adult circulation, such as erythrocytes, lymphocytes, monocytes, and neutrophil granulocytes. In naïve mice, neutrophils are produced and resisde in the BM extra-vascular compartment, where a large pool of mature neutrophils is stored, and part of the senescent neutrophils cleared. The liver and the spleen are also contributing to this clearance process. Mouse neutrophil generation/renewal, within steady state BM, takes place within myeloid islands centered on sialic acid-binding Ig-like lectin-1 (siglec-1) positive stromal macrophages. These islands support neutrophil granulocyte progenitor proliferation and differentiation [15]. Though the expression and features of siglec-1 could potentially influence many "macrophage-non macrophage cell interactions" in steady state, studies in siglec-1 deficient mice suggest that these interactions may be more important in the regulation of sustained T-dependent immune processes. As a result, there is a need to carry out experiments that combine genetic tools with high-resolution *in vivo* imaging in order to properly characterize the specific interactions that define the dynamic features of BM niches in steady state.

Of note, while the BM of a naïve mouse is estimated to store around 120 million neutrophils, the total number of neutrophils circulating in the blood vascular bed of a mouse is < 2.5 million. Within the BM reserve, mature neutrophils display low surface levels of CXCR4, but exhibit high intracellular levels of this receptor, suggesting that its ligand, SDF-1α/CXCL12, acts, in the BM, as a "retention" ligand for neutrophils. Once the mature neutrophils detach from their siglec-1 positive stromal macrophages, they interact with the VCAM-1, adhesion molecules constitutively displayed by BM sinusoidal endothelium. Though being displayed at low levels on mouse neutrophils, the α4β1 integrin accounts for the trans-endothelial migration of neutrophils across the VCAM-1 positive BM endothelium. In addition, HSPCs are themselves mobile and can continually traffic to other extra-medullary sites, such as the skin. There, if these HSPCs are sensing TLR agonists (endogenous as well as microbial) some of these HSPC will rapidly differentiate into mature myeloid cells. In summary, the non hematopoietic tissue at steady state is surveyed not only by resident cells but also by mobile HSPCs that home back to the BM as do pre-apoptotic senescent neutrophils [16, 17].

ACUTE INFLAMMATORY PROCESSES AND THEIR RAPID RESOLUTION WITHIN THE PIONEERING PERSPECTIVE OF METCHNIKOFF

An acute inflammatory process taking place in mammalian skin, consists of three components including: the inflammatory agonists, the sensors that detect them, the pro/counter inflammatory mediators released or synthesized as the results of the agonist/sensor interactions. Currently, four different classes of sensors have been identified: Germline encoded sensors that detect molecular features or patterns, *i.e.* Toll-like receptors (TLRs), C-type lectin receptors (CLRs), cytoplasmic proteins such as the Retinoic acid-inducible gene (RIG)-I-like receptors (RLRs), and NOD-like receptors (NLRs). These sensors are expressed not only in leukocytes but also in various non leukocyte lineages. Recent evidence indicates that in addition to microbial agonists, endogenous agonists can also be detected by these sensors. When a tissue is undergoing inflammatory processes, the inflammatory mediators act directly or indirectly on the tissue microvasculature inducing vasodilation, extravasation of neutrophils, and leakage of plasma into the extracellular matrix (ECM). The cytokine and chemokine profile in this inflammatory milieu will have elevated levels of mediators including IL-12p70, IL-12p40, TNF, TRAIL, IFNγ, IL-17 to IL-23.

In the absence of microbes, *i.e.*, in the case of sterile tissue injury, the damage is sensed by tissue damage sensors, and reparative processes are initiated by the rapid and synchronized clearance of apoptotic cells by macrophages or dendritic cells (DCs); it was shown that the ingestion of apoptotic cells such as neutrophils, triggers macrophages to release of TGF-β and IL-10 [18]. An inflammatory process may be prolonged by the G-CSF- or GM-CSF-dependent delay of neutrophil apoptosis, as well as by the lack of molecules such which are known to promote ingestion of apoptotic cells as the secreted glycoprotein milk fat globule-EGF-factor 8 (MFG-E8), TIM4 or stabilin-1 [19, 20]. Aside from the sustained presence of pro-inflammatory agonists, non resolution of inflammatory processes may result from deficiencies in the reparative mechanisms *per se* and from the unbalance of pro-inflammatory versus anti-inflammatory mediators.

The mammal skin, serves as a barrier between the body and the environment. Several cell lineages in the skin carry out key surveillance functions, including non hematopoietic lineages (epidermal, epithelial and dermal stromal cells), as well as hematopoietic cell lineages distributed in both the avascular epidermis and the vascularized sub-epidermal compartments.

THE NIMP-R14 mAB DISPLAYS FEATURES OF AN OPTIMAL REAGENT ALLOWING THE SELECTIVE, THOUGH TRANSIENT, DEPLETION OF MOUSE NEUTROPHILS *IN VIVO*

As briefly introduced above, neutrophils can contribute to phagocytosis and extracellular trap (ET) genesis to rapidly clear non opsonized and opsonized microbes. Neutrophils also interact with other cell lineages leading to the remodeling not only of the tissue, but also of the tissue-draining lymph node. Therefore, during acute or sustained inflammatory processes, neutrophils display a high plasticity that reflects 1) the features of the invasive microbe, 2) the onset of its development and 3) the tissue response that sense(s) some of the molecular patterns of the microbe as well as any other molecules co-delivered with the invasive microbe.

In mouse tissues experiencing either sterile injury or infection with microorganisms such as *Leishmania*, neutrophil functions need to be investigated with the proper approaches and/or reagents. Mice genetically engineered to exclusively target the neutrophil lineage functions still need to be developed, and antibodies that exclusively deplete the neutrophil lineage must be carefully characterized and their potential limitations considered.

The criteria used to identify mature mouse neutrophils have been based on the use of monoclonal antibody (mAb)-based reagents. The mAb, RB6-8C5 mAb [21], was shown to bind both Ly-6G and Ly-6C antigens [22]. This latter GPI-anchored molecule is also displayed on monocytes and dendritic cells. Thus, any immunological signatures observed after depletion with this antibody may not result solely from neutrophil depletion [23] making some interpretations of prior investigations performed with this antibody questionable [24-27].

Contrasting with the RB6-8C5 mAb, the 1A8 mAb could be used for neutrophil depletion. The 1A8 mAb has been obtained by fusion of myeloma rat cells with B cells recovered from rats to which the mouse Ly-6G protein was injected; this 1A8 mAb immunoprecipitates a protein of 21-25 kDa and binds exclusively to the Ly-6G protein used for immunization [22]. The limitation of the use of this mAb includes its partial *in vivo* depleting activity, and the need of a high dose of antibody to achieve depletion. Thus, the two former mAbs are not the ideal reagents to investigate processes strictly dependent upon neutrophils.

Therefore an antibody that combines specific recognition of neutrophils as well as good depleting efficiency *in vivo* would be useful. The NIMP-R14 mAb [28] has been obtained by injecting mouse BALB/c neutrophils into a rat; it cross-reacts with neutrophils from several mouse strains such as those of C57BL/6 mice. It precipitates a protein of 25-30 kDa. The NIMP-R14 mAb shows a good depleting efficiency *in vivo* and has been used as a neutrophil-depleting reagent to investigate the role of these leukocytes post *L. major* inoculation in mice [29-31]. However the exact epitope recognized by this mAb and its specificity for neutrophils have not been carefully investigated to date. Considering its good depleting efficiency, we went on to characterize its specificity and compared it to that of the two other neutrophil-depleting antibodies (RB6-8C5 and 1A8 mAbs).

We focused our studies on the recognition of the Ly-6G epitope, given that the protein precipitated with the NIMP-R14 mAb (25-30 kDa) was within the range of the Ly-6G protein (21-25 kDa). To this end, BM cells from C57BL/6 mice were stained with the RB6-8C5 (Ly-6G and Ly-6C), 1A8 (Ly-6G) or NIMP-R14 mAbs, with or without a pre-blocking step containing an excess of NIMP-R14 mAb. As shown in Fig. **1A**, staining of BM cells with both 1A8 and NIMP-R14 mAbs allows the discrimination of a double positive population corresponding to neutrophils (left panel). The pre-blocking step with the NIMP-R14 mAb resulted in the absence of binding of fluorescent NIMP-R14 mAb, confirming that all the recognition sites of NIMP-R14 were fully blocked (right panel). A population expressing low level of 1A8 still persisted after the NIMP-R14 pre-blocking step, indicating the existence of a partial overlapping epitope between the 1A8 and NIMP-R14 mAbs, and thus the recognition of Ly-6G by the NIMP-R14 mAb. BM cells stained with both the NIMP-R14 and RB6-8C5 mAbs (Fig. **1B**), revealed a different staining pattern as analyzed by FACS: 1) a double positive population that corresponds to the population of neutrophils displaying the Ly-6G epitope and 2) a RB6-8C5 single positive population that corresponds to a population of myeloid cells and their precursors displaying the Ly-6C epitope. When the pre-blocking step was performed with the NIMP- R14 mAb, the population that was double positive for RB6-8C5 and NIMP-R14 was not detectable and, similar to the 1A8 staining, a population expressing low level of RB6-8C5 expression persisted, while the single RB6-8C5 positive monocytes population remained unchanged. Similar results were obtained on BM cells of BALB/c mice (data not shown).

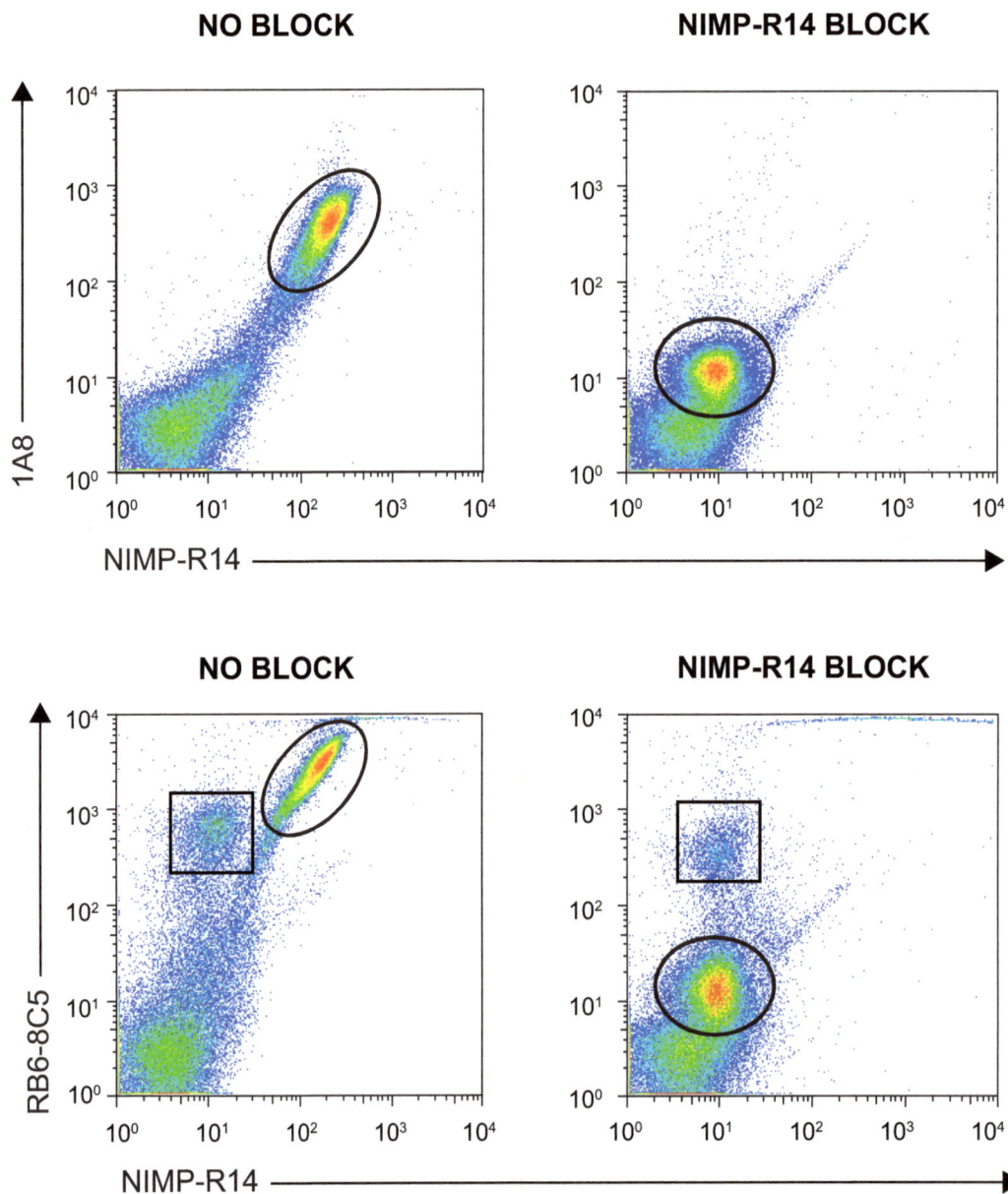

Figure 1: Phenotypic analysis of bone marrow cells allows sorting out the epitope(s) bound by the NIMP-R14 mAb. Naïve C57BL/6 mouse bone marrow cells were stained with the RB6-8C5, 1A8 or NIMP-R14 mAbs with (NIMP-R14 BLOCK) or without (NO BLOCK) pre-blocking with an excess of the NIMP-R14 mAb. The intenity of the staining was assessed by FACS. A. Co-staining with the 1A8 and NIMP-R14 mAb. B. Co-staining with the RB6-8C5 and NIMP-R14 mAbs. Data are representative of three independent experiments.

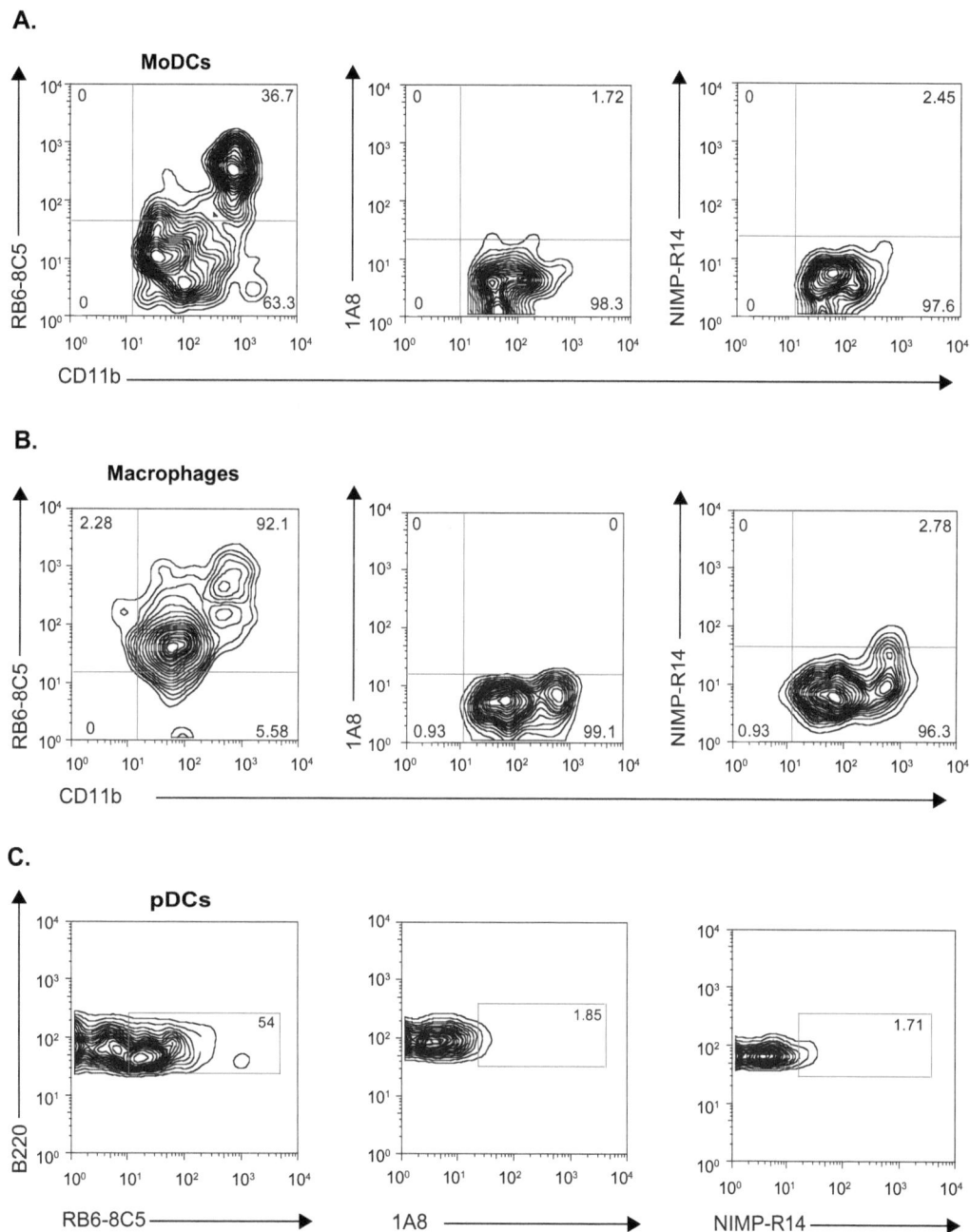

Figure 2: Contrasting with the RB6-8C5 mAb, the NIMP-R14 mAb exclusively binds to mouse neutrophils. (A.) Monocytes-derived dendritic cells gated as Ly-6G⁻ CD11b⁺ CD11c^{dim} and (B.) Macrophages gated as F4/80⁺ emigrating from ear explants 24 hours post *L. major* inoculation were incubated with the RB6-8C5, 1A8 and NIMP-R14 mAbs. C. Splenic plasmacytoid dendritic cells (CD3⁻ CD19⁻ F4/80⁻ CD11c⁺ B220⁺) were incubated with the RB6-8C5, 1A8 or NIMP-R14 mAbs. Data are representative of three independent experiments.

Altogether these data show that the NIMP-R14 mAb binds the neutrophil-specific Ly-6G epitopes-displaying protein, however the epitope recognized is shared but not identical to that recognized by the two other mAbs known to bind to the Ly-6G protein, or to this protein and its Ly-6C partner molecule. The different molecular weights (21-25 kDa for the 1A8 or RB6-8C5 mAbs vs. 25-30 kDa for the NIMP-R14 mAb) suggest some post-transcriptional modifications such as more or less extended glycosylation that might be recognized by the NIMP-R14 mAb. We next analyzed the recognition pattern of the three mAbs *ex vivo*. To this end, we used the technique of ear explants [32-34]. Briefly, *L. major* stationary phase promastigotes were given intradermally into the C57BL/6 mouse ear dermis, and the ears were recovered 24 hours later. Dorsal and ventral sheets of the ears were separated, the dermal side was placed down on medium for sedimentation. The leukocytes emigrating over 24 hours were collected for further analysis. We examined monocyte-derived dendritic cells (MoDCs), macrophages, and plasmacytoid dendritic cells (pDCs) as these cells are recognized by the RB6-8C5 mAb through the Ly-6C molecule shared by these subsets. MoDCs were characterized by FACS as being Ly-6G$^-$ CD11b$^+$ CD11c^{dim}. As shown in Fig. **2A**, the MoDC population was recognized neither by the NIMP-R14 mAb nor by the 1A8 mAb, while staining with the RB6-8C5 mAb revealed a clear population of MoDCs (Fig. **2A**, left panel). We next analyzed the emigrating leukocyte populations for the presence of macrophages, the latter being identified by the F4/80 mAb. As shown in Fig. **2B**, the RB6-8C5 mAb recognized macrophages, while the 1A8 and NIMP-R14 mAbs did not stain these cells. A small population (2-3%) of F4/80$^+$ CD11b$^+$ Ly-6C^{hi} CD11c$^-$ was weakly stained with the NIMP-R14 mAb. Plasmacytoid DCs (pDCs) have been shown to bind the RB6-8C5 mAb. Since only a low number of pDCs were recruited shortly after intradermal inoculation of *L. major*, we used a spleen from a naïve C57BL/6 mouse to visualize pDCs. The pDCs population was characterized by FACS as being CD3$^-$ CD19$^-$ F4/80$^-$ CD11c$^+$ B220$^+$. While this pDC population was stained with the RB6-8C5 mAb (Fig. **2C**, left panel), it was not bound neither by the NIMP-R14 mAb (Fig. **2C**, right panel) nor the 1A8 mAb (Fig. **2C**, middle panel). Thus, together with recent data published [23, 35, 36], our data establish that the CD11b$^+$ Gr-1^{hi} cells in mouse BM, or in the leukocyte population emigrating from *Leishmania*-infected ears can be clearly separated into two populations according to Ly-6G expression. While both 1A8 and NIMP-R14 mAbs bind a surface molecule that is specific to mouse neutrophils, the optimal reagent to deplete neutrophils *in vivo* is the NIMP-R14 mAb.

WHEN THE MOUSE SKIN EXPERIENCES A "NON SILENT" ENTRY OF *L. major*, THE MATURE NEUTROPHIL POPULATION CAN CONTRIBUTE TO THE ONSET OF THE *L. major*-SPECIFIC IMMUNE RESPONSE

Upon transmission of *L. major* metacyclic promastigotes by sand flies or with a syringe (high doses of stationary phase promastigotes delivered in the dermis), neutrophils are known to be rapidly recruited to the site of *L. major* inoculation. According to the mouse strain features, the duration of neutrophil recruitment, and the partition of neutrophils between the *L. major*-loaded skin and the skin-draining lymph node were shown to differ over the first days post parasite inoculation. This will have an impact on the subsequent distinct phases that 1) either proceed from a clinically silent phase to a transient lesion followed by tissue repair or 2) proceed from a clinically silent phase to a non healing prolonged lesion (reviewed in [37-39]).

Considering that neutrophils rapidly exit their BM storage compartment to reach the skin site of *L. major* inoculation, they may be an important source of signals that contribute to the microenvironment found at the parasite inoculation site. Therefore, the understanding of the factors controlling neutrophil persistence at the site of inoculation is of importance not only for parasite control but also in immune regulation. When comparing the neutrophil recruitment at the *L. major* inoculated site in BALB/c and C57BL/6 mice, there are qualitative and quantitative differences observed from three days post parasite inoculation, with characteristics of a sustained neutrophil-rich inflammatory process in BALB/c mice, whereas in C57BL/6 mice, macrophages become the predominant cell population with only a low number of neutrophils remaining locally [29, 40, 41]. At these early time points, when the *Leishmania* triggered processes is initiated, other features than the mammal genotype also account for the distinct composition of the leukocyte infiltrates at the site of inoculation. Briefly, when sand fly salivary gland extract are co-inoculated with high dose of *Leishmania* promastigotes, a higher number of intracellular amastigotes was detected, in parallel with a sustained neutrophil recruitment [42]. More recently, *Leishmania*-hosting *Phlebotomus dubosqi* were used to inoculate parasites mimicking its natural entry. A low number of metacyclic promastigotes was co-delivered with both sand fly saliva and promastigotes derived filamentous PPG into the C57BL/6 mouse dermis [24]. With this model, it became possible to compare syringe-dependent *L. major* inoculation to sand fly-dependent inoculation. While the neutrophils were no more detectable three days post parasite injection following syringe injection, neutrophils were, in contrast, dominating the leukocyte infiltrates over eight days post infection with *Leishmania*-loaded sand flies [31]. Thus, the control of neutrophil clearance at the site of parasite inoculation depends on multiple factors derived both from the mammal host and from the sand fly. Of note, when the *Leishmania*-hosting sand fly is only probing the mouse skin, only a low number of immediately motile metacyclic promastigotes are co-delivered in the dermis with a small amount of saliva; in contrast, when the *Leishmania*-hosting sand fly is successfully taking its blood meal a higher number of metacyclic promastigotes are regurgitated with both saliva and PPG within a blood pool. The importance of these factors were recently highlighted in mice vaccinated with a heat killed *Leishmania* vaccine (autoclaved *L. major* plus CpG oligodeoxynucleotide) where lesion did not develop following syringe-based *Leishmania* inoculation; however, in mice similarly vaccinated but infected by sand flies, lesions developed. Interestingly, if the vaccinated mice where depleted of neutrophils prior to the sand fly-based *Leishmania* inoculation, they did not display any lesion [31]. These results further support the need for a better understanding of neutrophil functions in local and downstream sites, such as the skin-draining lymph nodes to more distant tissues such as the liver, the spleen and the BM.

Following *Leishmania* inoculation, in addition to the phagocytosis and NET functions displayed by neutrophils, these cells release specific molecules that account for the recruitment of other leukocyte subsets. When exposed to *Leishmania* metacyclic promastigotes, neutrophils have been shown to release/secrete immune mediators such as cytokines and chemokines that could shape the developing immune response. In this line, it was reported that at the site of *L. major* inoculation, C57BL/6 neutrophils secreted biologically active IL-12p70 and IL-10. In contrast, BALB/c neutrophils transcribed and secreted high levels of IL-12p40 but did not secrete biologically active IL-12p70. Furthermore, this IL-12p40 did not associate with IL-23p19, but formed IL-12p40 homodimers with inhibitory activity. In addition, after their co-incubation with *L. major* metacyclic promastigotes, BALB/c mouse BM neutrophils secreted TGF-β but did not secrete IL-10 [43]. Uptake of dying neutrophils by macrophages was shown to elicit distinct secretion of cytokines by C57BL/6 vs. BALB/c macrophages with BALB/c macrophages secreting TGF-β, promoting parasite growth; while C57BL/6 neutrophils secreted TNF and elastase, both molecules conferring leishmanicidal activity to macrophages [26].

Thus following inoculation of *L. major,* distinct neutrophil phenotypes are observed in different mouse strains: in C57BL/6 mice, neutrophils could constitute one of the earliest sources of bioactive IL-12, while in BALB/c mice, secretion of IL-12p40 could contribute to impairment of early IL-12 signaling. In addition, interaction with other leukocytes such as resident macrophages, monocytes, and dendritic cells (DCs) present at the site of parasite inoculation may impact the early cytokine/chemokine milieu, thereby influencing the outcome of the parasite-hosting dermal site. Altogether, these results indicate that the distinct neutrophil phenotypes observed following infection with *L. major* might influence the *L. major*-reactive T-dependent immune response *in vivo.* With respect to the latter immune processes, one of the most significant outcomes of the cross talk occurring among leukocytes present or recruited at the site of inoculation will be the effects on DCs, the leukocytes programmed to deliver within the skin-draining lymph node, immunogenic information that results in the activation of balanced or unbalanced population of pro-inflammatory effector T lymphocytes or inflammation. The role of neutrophils in the recruitment of immature DCs has been recently documented in mice inoculated with a high dose of *L. major* stationary promastigotes. The secretion of DC-attracting chemokines varied significantly in *L. major*-exposed BALB/c vs. C57BL/6 neutrophils. While in presence of *L. major,* BALB/c neutrophils secrete very low chemokine amounts, a significant secretion of CCL3 (macrophage inflammatory protein 1 alpha, MIP-1α) is released by C57BL/6 neutrophils both *in vitro* and *ex vivo* [34]. The CCL3 released by C57BL/6 neutrophils exposed to *L. major* metacyclic promastigotes was further shown to be responsible for the early chemoattraction of DCs to the site of parasite inoculation. Depletion of neutrophils or the transient neutralization of CCL3 over the first days post parasite inoculation resulted in a marked decrease of the DCs as well as the monocyte-derived DCs emigrating from the *L. major*-loaded ear explants. The defective mobilization of DCs measured in mice genetically deficient in CCL3 could be corrected by the simultaneous injection of wild type neutrophils with parasites at the site of parasite inoculation, revealing the crucial role of neutrophil-secreted CCL3 in DC recruitment. The decrease in DC number had an immunological impact at early time points post *L. major* inoculation. Indeed, neutralization of CCL3 during the first days following parasite inoculation had a marked, though transient, effect on the development of a CD4+ Th1 type of immune response, decreasing the secretion of IFNγ by CD4+ T cells during the first weeks post parasite inoculation [34].

PERSPECTIVES

Altogether, several recent studies have emphasized the previously underappreciated role of neutrophils as players in the remodeling of the skin and its skin-draining lymph node as a long term niche where parasites develop. Neutrophils first play a role in sheltering and shuttling of promastigotes, features addressed in other chapters, and second, through their release of constitutive and inducible cytokines and chemokines, the latter allowing subsequent dialogs with other non neutrophil leukocyte subsets. When comparing C57BL/6 and BALB/c mice inoculated with cultured stationary phase promastigotes two distinct outcomes were reported: in C57BL/6 mice the *Leishmania*-protective and skin-protective niches can be remodeled independently from the contribution of the early neutrophil wave, while BALB/c mice exhibit sustained skin-damaging processes taking place at the *L. major* inoculation site, possibly reflecting the lack of CCL3-chemoattracted DC subsets at the onset of the intracellular amastigote population amplification phase. These contrasting features need to be further explored at both the level of neutrophils and within the frame of their transient interactions with many other cell lineages cooperating in the wounded skin both at the time of parasite delivery, and over the first hours post parasite delivery. In addition, as distinct *L. major* isolates as well as different *Leishmania* species have been reported to differentially contribute to skin remodeling at the site of infection [44], it would be of interest to investigate whether neutrophils will still be one of the major early contributors following infection with other *Leishmania* species. Finally, the present data are strong incentives to further explore the early processes deployed in wild rodent skin, when a *Leishmania*-hosting sand fly has deposited metacyclic promastigotes either in presence of saliva in a minimally wounded skin, or in presence of saliva and parasite derived PPG in the blood pool in an extensively wounded skin. Recent studies have highlighted the importance of keratinocytes as sensors of steady state-disruptive signals and of bidirectional traffic of regulatory T lymphocytes [45-47]. Together with the functions highlighted in the present chapter, these recently identified functions reflect how signals initiating and terminating inflammatory processes must be tightly controlled, and how *Leishmania* perpetuation relies on these multilayered processes.

MATERIAL AND METHODS

Leishmania major Promastigote Inoculum, Mice and intradermal Inoculation

L. major (LV 39 MRHO/Sv/59/P strain) were maintained, grown and the inoculum of stationary phase promastigotes were prepared as previously described [48]. Female C57BL/6 mice were purchased from Harlan Olac Ltd. (Bicester, UK). Mice were bred in the pathogen-free facility at the BIL Epalinges Center and used at 6 weeks of age and were given intradermally, into one of their two ears, 10^6 stationary phase *L. major* promastigotes. All mouse-based explorations were approved by the veterinary office regulations of the State of Vaud, Switzerland, authorization 1266.3 to FTC, and experiments were performed adhering to protocols created by this office.

Ear Explant Model

Mouse ears collected 24 hours post L. major inoculation were processed as previously described [32], with the ear ventral and dorsal sheets being separated with forceps and the two leaflets being transferred dermal side down in a plate containing RPMI-1640 media supplemented with 10% FCS and antibiotics at 37°C. The leukocyte populations spontaneously emigrating, over 14 hours, from these ear leaflets/explants were then counted and stained for FACS analysis.

Splenocyte Population Preparation

The spleen from C57BL/6 mice was digested using with a mix a DNAse (1 mg/ml) and Collagenase D (0.5 mg/ml) and incubated 30 minutes at 37°C. It was further homogenized, and cells were stained with the indicated mAbs.

FACS Analysis of the Single Cell Populations

Cells were processed for cell surface staining. The mAb 24G2 was used to block FcRs. For the different staining several mAbs were used: FITC conjugated NIMP-R14 mAb [28], FITC and PE conjugated anti-Ly-6G (clone 1A8), Cyc conjugated anti-CD11c (clone N418), FITC conjugated anti-Ly-6C (clone AL-21), Cyc conjugated anti-CD11b (clone M1/70), all mAbs from e-Bioscience, SanDiego, CA, US. Biotinylated anti-F4/80 (clone C1:A3-1, CEDARLANE, Canada). Cells were analyzed with a FACScan (3 colors) or FACSCalibur (4 colors) (BD Biosciences, Mountain View, CA, USA) and analyzed using the program FlowJo (Tree Star. Inc., Ashland, OR, USA).

ACKNOWLEDGEMENT

We thank Dr T. Weinkopff for critical reading of the manuscript. This work was supported by grants to FTC from the Swiss National Science Foundation (320000-116197).

REFERENCES

[1]   Ashford RW. The *leishmaniases* as emerging and reemerging zoonoses. Int J Parasitol 2000; 30(12-13):1269-81.

[2]   Desjeux P. *Leishmania*sis: current situation and new perspectives. Comp Immunol Microbiol Infect Dis 2004; 27(5):305-18.

[3]   Gramiccia M, Gradoni L. The current status of zoonotic *leishmaniases* and approaches to disease control. Int J Parasitol 2005; 35(11-12):1169-80.

[4]   Murray HW, Berman JD, Davies CR, Saravia NG. Advances in *leishmaniasis*. Lancet 2005; 366(9496):1561-77.

[5]   Bern C, Maguire JH, Alvar J. Complexities of assessing the disease burden attributable to *leishmania*sis. PLoS Negl Trop Dis 2008; 2(10):e313.

[6]   Reithinger R. *Leishmaniases*' burden of disease: ways forward for getting from speculation to reality. PLoS Negl Trop Dis 2008; 2(10):e285.

[7]   Rogers ME, Chance ML, Bates PA. The role of promastigote secretory gel in the origin and transmission of the infective stage of *Leishmania mexicana* by the sandfly Lutzomyia longipalpis. Parasitology 2002; 124(Pt 5):495-507.

[8]   Rogers ME, Ilg T, Nikolaev AV, Ferguson MA, Bates PA. Transmission of cutaneous *leishmaniasis* by sand flies is enhanced by regurgitation of fPPG. Nature 2004; 430(6998):463-7.

[9]   Volf P, Hajmova M, Sadlova J, Votypka J. Blocked stomodeal valve of the insect vector: similar mechanism of transmission in two trypanosomatid models. Int J Parasitol 2004; 34(11):1221-7.

[10] Bates PA, Rogers ME. New insights into the developmental biology and transmission mechanisms of *Leishmania*. Curr Mol Med 2004; 4(6):601-9.

[11] Kamhawi S. Phlebotomine sand flies and *Leishmania* parasites: friends or foes? Trends Parasitol 2006; 22(9):439-45.

[12] Bates PA. Transmission of *Leishmania* metacyclic promastigotes by phlebotomine sand flies. Int J Parasitol 2007; 37(10):1097-106.

[13] Jaiswal S, Weissman IL. Hematopoietic stem and progenitor cells and the inflammatory response. Ann N Y Acad Sci 2009; 1174:118-21.

[14] Schulz C, von Andrian UH, Massberg S. Hematopoietic stem and progenitor cells: their mobilization and homing to bone marrow and peripheral tissue. Immunol Res 2009; 44(1-3):160-8.

[15] Crocker PR, Redelinghuys P. Siglecs as positive and negative regulators of the immune system. Biochem Soc Trans 2008; 36(Pt 6):1467-71.

[16] Furze RC, Rankin SM. Neutrophil mobilization and clearance in the bone marrow. Immunology 2008; 125(3):281-8.

[17] Massberg S, von Andrian UH. Novel trafficking routes for hematopoietic stem and progenitor cells. Ann N Y Acad Sci 2009; 1176:87-93.

[18] Kennedy AD, DeLeo FR. Neutrophil apoptosis and the resolution of infection. Immunol Res 2009; 43(1-3):25-61.

[19] Rossi AG, Hallett JM, Sawatzky DA, Teixeira MM, Haslett C. Modulation of granulocyte apoptosis can influence the resolution of inflammation. Biochem Soc Trans 2007; 35(Pt 2):288-91.

[20] Fox S, Leitch AE, Duffin R, Haslett C, Rossi AG. Neutrophil Apoptosis: Relevance to the innate immune response Ans Inflammatory Disease. J Innate Immun 2010.

[21] Hestdal K, Ruscetti FW, Ihle JN, *et al.* Characterization and regulation of RB6-8C5 antigen expression on murine bone marrow cells. J Immunol 1991; 147(1):22-8.

[22] Fleming TJ, O'HUigin C, Malek TR. Characterization of two novel Ly-6 genes. Protein sequence and potential structural similarity to alpha-bungarotoxin and other neurotoxins. J Immunol 1993; 150(12):5379-90.

[23] Zhang X, Majlessi L, Deriaud E, Leclerc C, Lo-Man R. Coactivation of Syk kinase and MyD88 adaptor protein pathways by bacteria promotes regulatory properties of neutrophils. Immunity 2009; 31(5):761-71.

[24] Peters NC, Egen JG, Secundino N, *et al. In vivo* imaging reveals an essential role for neutrophils in *leishmaniasis* transmitted by sand flies. Science 2008 ; 321(5891):970-4.

[25] Lima GM, Puel A, Decreusefond C, *et al.* Susceptibility and resistance to *Leishmania amazonensis* in H-2q syngeneic high and low antibody responder mice (Biozzi mice). Scand J Immunol 1998; 48(2):144-51.

[26] Ribeiro-Gomes FL, Otero AC, Gomes NA, *et al.* Macrophage interactions with neutrophils regulate *Leishmania major* infection. J Immunol 2004; 172(7):4454-62.

[27] Chen L, Zhang ZH, Watanabe T, *et al.* The involvement of neutrophils in the resistance to *Leishmania major* infection in susceptible but not in resistant mice. Parasitol Int 2005; 54(2):109-18.

[28] Lopez AF, Strath M, Sanderson CJ. Differentiation antigens on mouse eosinophils and neutrophils identified by monoclonal antibodies. Br J Haematol 1984; 57(3):489-94.

[29] Tacchini-Cottier F, Zweifel C, Belkaid Y, *et al.* An immunomodulatory function for neutrophils during the induction of a CD4+ Th2 response in BALB/c mice infected with *Leishmania major*. J Immunol 2000; 165(5):2628-36.

[30] McFarlane E, Perez C, Charmoy M, *et al.* Neutrophils contribute to development of a protective immune response during onset of infection with *Leishmania donovani.* Infect Immun 2008;76(2):532-41.

[31] Peters NC, Kimblin N, Secundino N, Kamhawi S, Lawyer P, Sacks DL. Vector transmission of *leishmania* abrogates vaccine-induced protective immunity. PLoS Pathog 2009; 5(6):e1000484.

[32] Belkaid Y, Jouin H, Milon G. A method to recover, enumerate and identify lymphomyeloid cells present in an inflammatory dermal site: a study in laboratory mice. J Immunol Methods 1996; 199(1):5-25.

[33] Belkaid Y, Mendez S, Lira R, Kadambi N, Milon G, Sacks D. A natural model of *Leishmania major* infection reveals a prolonged "silent" phase of parasite amplification in the skin before the onset of lesion formation and immunity. J Immunol 2000 ;165(2):969-77.

[34] Charmoy M, Brunner-Agten S, Aebischer D, *et al.* Neutrophil-Derived CCL3 Is Essential for the Rapid Recruitment of Dendritic Cells to the Site of *Leishmania major* Inoculation in Resistant Mice. PLoS Pathog 2010;6(2):e1000755.

[35] Daley JM, Thomay AA, Connolly MD, Reichner JS, Albina JE. Use of Ly6G-specific monoclonal antibody to deplete neutrophils in mice. J Leukoc Biol 2008; 83(1):64-70.

[36] Abbitt KB, Cotter MJ, Ridger VC, Crossman DC, Hellewell PG, Norman KE. Antibody ligation of murine Ly-6G induces neutropenia, blood flow cessation, and death via complement-dependent and independent mechanisms. J Leukoc Biol 2009; 85(1):55-63.

[37] Peters NC, Sacks DL. The impact of vector-mediated neutrophil recruitment on cutaneous *leishmaniasis.* Cell Microbiol 2009; 11(9):1290-6.

[38] Charmoy M, Auderset F, Allenbach C, Tacchini-Cottier F. The prominent role of neutrophils during the initial phase of infection by *Leishmania* parasites. J Biomed Biotechnol 2010; 719361.

[39] Ritter U, Frischknecht F, van Zandbergen G. Are neutrophils important host cells for *Leishmania* parasites? Trends Parasitol 2009; 25(11):505-10.

[40] Beil WJ, Meinardus-Hager G, Neugebauer DC, Sorg C. Differences in the onset of the inflammatory response to cutaneous *leishmania*sis in resistant and susceptible mice. J Leukoc Biol 1992; 52(2):135-42.

[41] Allenbach C, Launois P, Mueller C, Tacchini-Cottier F. An essential role for transmembrane TNF in the resolution of the inflammatory lesion induced by *Leishmania major* infection. Eur J Immunol 2008; 38(3):720-31.

[42] Donnelly KB, Lima HC, Titus RG. Histologic characterization of experimental cutaneous *leishmania*sis in mice infected with *Leishmania braziliensis* in the presence or absence of sand fly vector salivary gland lysate. J Parasitol 1998; 84(1):97-103.

[43] Charmoy M, Megnekou R, Allenbach C, *et al. Leishmania major* induces distinct neutrophil phenotypes in mice that are resistant or susceptible to infection. J Leukoc Biol 2007; 82(2):288-99.

[44] Revaz-Breton M, Ronet C, Ives A, *et al.* MyD88 pathway is differently involved in immune responses induced by distinct substrains of *Leishmania major.* Eur J Immunol.

[45] Nestle FO, Di Meglio P, Qin JZ, Nickoloff BJ. Skin immune sentinels in health and disease. Nat Rev Immunol 2009; 9(10):679-91.

[46] Matsushima H, Takashima A. Bidirectional homing of Tregs between the skin and lymph nodes. J Clin Invest;120(3):653-6.

[47] Ehrchen JM, Roebrock K, Foell D, *et al.* Keratinocytes determine Th1 immunity during early experimental *leishmaniasis.* PLoS Pathog 2010; 6(4):e1000871.

[48] Louis J, Moedder E, Behin R, Engers H. Recognition of protozoan parasite antigens by murine T lymphocytes. I. Induction of specific T lymphocyte-dependent proliferative response to *Leishmania tropica.* Eur J Immunol 1979; 9(11):841-7.

CHAPTER 7

Understanding Neutrophil Function During *Toxoplasma gondii* Infection

Eric Y. Denkers[*]

Department of Microbiology and Immunology, College of Veterinary Medicine, Cornell University, Ithaca, NY 14853-6401 USA

Abstract: Neutrophils are the most common type of leukocyte. They are produced in large number by the bone marrow and they rapidly accumulate at sites of invasion by microbial pathogens, including the opportunistic protozoan parasite *Toxoplasma gondii*. Here, current data on the role of neutrophils during *T. gondii* infection are reviewed. On the one hand, neutrophils may play a role in facilitating establishment of a stable host-parasite interaction. They may maximize the probability of parasite transmission by promoting an effective immune response that enables both host survival and establishment of persistent infection. On the other hand, these cells may be important purely for the host by acting as potent destroyers of parasites. Collateral tissue damage may be the unavoidable consequence.

INTRODUCTION

Biology and Immunology of *Toxoplasma* Infection

The protozoan *Toxoplasma gondii* is a commonly occurring parasite in human and animal populations worldwide. Up to 30-50% of the human population is estimated to be chronically infected with this microorganism [1]. Although in most cases infection is asymptomatic, in immunocompromised populations the parasite emerges as a life-threatening pathogen causing toxoplasmic encephalitis [2]. Congenital infection with *Toxoplasma* can also have extremely serious consequences to the developing fetus, including blindness, mental retardation and death [3].

Infection is initiated by ingestion of tissue cysts or oocysts shed by cats [1]. In the small intestine, the parasite differentiates into rapidly replicating tachyzoites that invade cells and establish residence in a specialized parasitophorous vacuole. Within this niche, tachyzoites replicate and eventually egress from host cells [4]. The parasite disseminates via the blood and lymph to infect a wide range of host tissues [5]. With the rise in adaptive immunity, tachyzoites differentiate into slow growing bradyzoites that form quiescent cysts in tissues of the skeletal muscle and central nervous system. The parasite can persist in this form for the lifetime of the host as an asymptomatic infection. Yet, *T. gondii* is an opportunistic infection insofar as an intact immune system is required to maintain the parasite in this quiescent state [6-8]. *Toxoplasma* replicates asexually for most of its life cycle in most host species. However, for reasons that remain unknown infection in the cat intestine results in a sexual reproductive phase of the parasite culminating in shedding of highly infectious oocysts in the feces [1].

Toxoplasma is a prototypic Th1 inducing pathogen [9]. Infection is marked by high levels of IL-12 and IFN-γ, and in mice these cytokines are required for survival during both acute and chronic infection [8, 10-12]. In addition to $CD4^+$ Th1 lymphocytes, $CD8^+$ T cell effectors play a protective role through IFN-γ production and cytolytic activity [13, 14]. One function of IFN-γ is thought to be through induction of inducible nitric oxide synthase (iNOS) resulting in nitric oxide (NO)-mediated killing, particularly during chronic infection [15]. In addition, IFN-γ induces a family of immunity-related GTPase (IRG) proteins that disassemble the parasitophorous vacuole causing death of the parasite, a mechanism that is particularly important during acute infection [16].

Despite the importance of IFN-γ for protection, *Toxoplasma* can also cause proinflammatory pathology in certain circumstances and it is important that production of this cytokine is tightly controlled. The cytokine IL-10 plays a key role in preventing overproduction of proinflammatory mediators during *T. gondii* infection [17-19]. Nevertheless, certain virulent parasite strains (the so-called Type I strains) trigger uncontrolled proinflammatory responses in mice that result in early mortality [20, 21]. Furthermore, some inbred mice (for example, the C57BL/6 strain) are prone to intestinal immunopathology during oral infection [22]. Emerging evidence suggests that this may be triggered by changes in the endogenous gut flora rather than *Toxoplasma* itself [23-25].

Address correspondence to Eric Y. Denkers at: Department of Microbiology and Immunology, College of Veterinary Medicine, Cornell University, Ithaca, NY 14853-6401 USA; E-mail: eyd1@cornell.edu

Fabienne Tacchini-Cottier and Ger van Zandbergen (Eds)

A major aspect of the host-parasite interaction for *T. gondii* is the parasite's encounter with the innate immune system. Toll-like receptor (TLR) signaling pathways play a key role in early recognition of infection, as demonstrated by the extreme susceptibility of MyD88 knockout mice [26-28]. In this regard, a parasite profilin molecule has been identified as a ligand of TLR11 [29, 30], and tachyzoite glycosylinositol phospholipid moieties are reported to activate TLR2 and TLR4 [31]. There is also evidence that TLR9 plays a role during *T. gondii* infection, although the relevant ligands in this case have not been identified [32, 33].

Dendritic cells are important initiators of immunity through IL-12 production, and indeed there is evidence that this cell type is actively targeted for infection by *T. gondii* [5, 34-36]. Macrophages, in particular Gr-1$^+$ inflammatory macrophages, are believed to be important microbicidal effector cells [37, 38]. As described in the following sections, there is also evidence that neutrophils are an important component in the immune response to infection, although their precise role is still uncertain.

Toxoplasma-Neutrophil Interactions: *in vitro* Studies

Neutrophils are classically regarded as microbicidal effector cells that provide a first line of defense against infection. This is mediated by multiple factors, including production of reactive oxygen intermediates, the enzymatic activity of neutrophil granule contents, and more recently the production of neutrophil extracellular traps (NET). Older studies suggest that human peripheral blood neutrophils are capable of killing parasites, particularly if they are opsonized [39-41], although the mechanisms involved in parasiticidal function have not been addressed. Despite apparent killing activity, it is also clear from *in vitro* [40, 42] and *in vivo* (our unpublished observations) studies that *Toxoplasma* is capable of establishing residence in polymorphonuclear leukocytes (PMN), although neutrophils are less permissive to parasite replication compared to cells such as macrophages and fibroblasts. Regardless, this raises the possibility that PMN play a Trojan horse role for *Toxoplasma*, particularly since these cells accumulate in draining lymph nodes during infection which seems to be a major route of parasite dissemination [28].

There is clear evidence that PMN serve as a source of multiple cytokines during infection [43-45]. On a per cell basis, they tend to produce less cytokine than cells such as macrophages and dendritic cells. Nevertheless, the ability of neutrophils to accumulate in high number at sites of infection and inflammation suggests that these cells may be a highly significant source of cytokines on a population basis. We found that mouse PMN produce several cytokines and chemokines after stimulation with *Toxoplasma* soluble antigen, including IL-12p40 that is key in the host response to infection (Table **1**) [46, 47]. Furthermore, IL-12 appears to be expressed in preformed stores in neutrophils [48]. In line with this observation, PMN have also been reported to express IL-6, CXC chemokine-2 (CXCL2/MIP-2) and IL-4 as preformed pools of cytokine [49-51]. Thus, neutrophils appear to be specialized to rapidly release cytokines without the need for de novo protein synthesis. Nevertheless, in addition to evidence that PMN emerge from the bone marrow with preformed cytokine, these cells can upregulate cytokine gene transcription in response to *ex vivo* stimulation, at least for the case of IL-12 and MIP-2 [48, 50]. It is also apparent that human PMN produce IL-12p40 as well as TNF-α in response to *Toxoplasma*. Interestingly, TNF-α appears to act in autocrine fashion to induce neutrophil production of CC chemokine ligand (CCL)-3 and CCL4 [46].

Table 1: Cytokines and chemokines produced by neutrophils after *Toxoplasma* stimulation.

Cytokine/Chemokine	Live vs. STAg[1]	PMNsource[2]
IL-12p40	Live, STAg	Human; mouse
TNF-α	Live, STAg	Human; mouse
CCL2/MCP-1	Live, STAg	Mouse
CCL3/MIP-1α	Live, STAg	Human; mouse
CCL4/MIP-1β	Live, STAg	Human; mouse
CCL5/RANTES	Live	Mouse
CCL20/MIP-3α	Live	Mouse

[1]Live, cells cultured with live tachyzoites; STAg, cells cultured with soluble tachyzoite antigen (STAg). [2]PMN purified from human peripheral blood or from mouse peritoneal cavity following thioglycollate elicitation.

When neutrophil IL-12p40 and CCL2 were examined in the mouse model, we found that the responses were regulated differently [52]. Thus, partial biochemical fractionation of parasite soluble antigen revealed that the molecules inducing IL-12p40 and CCL2 were distinct. Although both activities were MyD88 dependent, the CCL2 but not the IL-12 response required TLR2. Of further interest, IL-10 was a potent suppressor of neutrophil IL-12p40, but it had no effect on parasite antigen-induced CCL2. IFN-γ/STAT1 signaling increased production of both IL-12p40 and CCL2 in response to *T. gondii*. For CCL2, IFN-γ/STAT1 alone induced expression. However production of both IL-12p40 and CCL2 required signaling through the JNK2 mitogen-activated protein kinase [53]. Thus, with regard to PMN (and most likely other cell types), there is a complexity in MyD88-dependent signaling to microbial antigen, in that multiple signaling pathways leading to distinct outcomes can simultaneously be triggered after upstream receptor-ligand binding (Fig. 1).

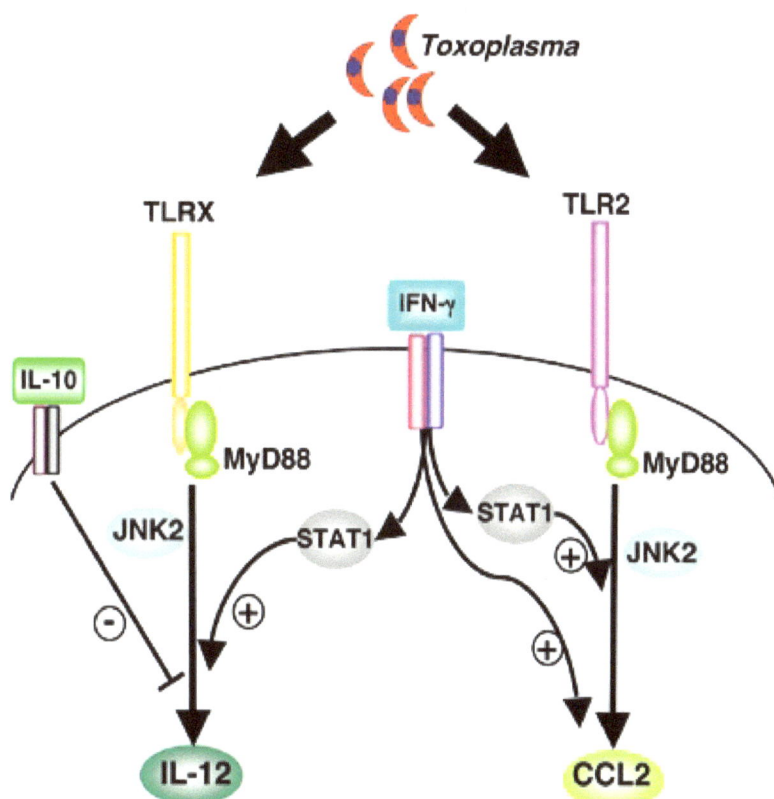

Figure 1: Control of *T. gondii*-triggered IL-12 and CCL2 production by neutrophils. A tachyzoite-derived factor triggers MyD88- and JNK2-dependent IL-12 through an unidentified TLR. The pathway is sensitive to Stat1-dependent IFN-γ-mediated upregulation. Signaling mediated by anti-inflammatory cytokine IL-10 down-regulates this signaling cascade. A distinct parasite factor triggers neutrophil CCL2 production in dependence upon TLR2, MyD88 and JNK2. This pathway is insensitive to IL-10. IFN-γ alone upregulates CCL2 production in a STAT1-independent manner. In combination with the parasite, the effects of IFN-γ display a partial dependence on STAT1, suggesting that, in addition to direct effects on CCL2 induction, IFN-γ acts through STAT1 to upregulate the *T. gondii* triggered pathway leading to CCL2 production.

In addition to release of cytokines such as IL-12 that can polarize T cell differentiation, there is evidence that neutrophils can instruct DC activation, in turn promoting Th1 differentiation [54]. *Toxoplasma* triggers neutrophil release of CCL3, CCL4, CCL5 and CCL20. These chemokines act as strong chemoattractants of immature DC. PMN incubated with tachyzoites release factors that induce costimulatory molecule expression and high-level IL-12p40 and TNF-α production by bone marrow-derived DC [55]. This is in part due to TNF-α release by stimulated neutrophils themselves. Remarkably similar findings have been reported by others using human DC and PMN. In that case, direct interaction between DC-SIGN with Lewis[x] carbohydrates on neutrophil Mac-1 and CEACAM1 are required to induce DC maturation [56, 57]. A plausible model suggested by these studies is that neutrophils recruited to sites of infection release chemokines that in turn attract DC. Interactions between PMN and DC could then result in activation of the latter, contributing to the triggering of adaptive immunity [54, 58]. A similar model has recently been proposed during *Leishmania major* infection [59].

In vivo Studies

While it is clear that neutrophils respond to *Toxoplasma* during *in vitro* infection, less is known about their role after infection *in vivo* (Fig. **2**). Thus, the degree to which they function as direct killers, whether they also play a role in orchestrating DC function, and their contribution to inflammatory pathology is not so clear.

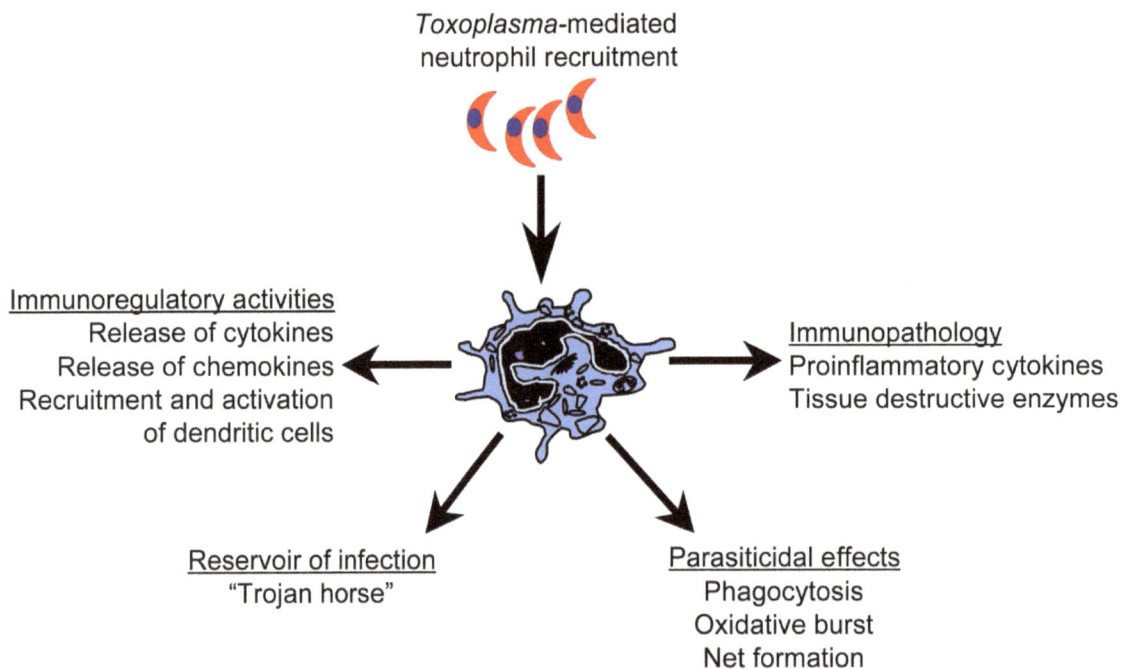

Figure 2: Potential roles for neutrophils during *Toxoplasma* infection. Neutrophils are rapidly recruited to sites of infection dependent upon CXCR2 and MyD88. The cells may respond to infection by releasing chemokines and cytokines that recruit and activate other cells of the immune system. *In vitro* studies suggest dendritic cells are targets of neutrophil-derived immunoregulatory cytokines and chemokines. *Toxoplasma* is also capable of infecting neutrophils. Accumulation of PMN in draining lymph nodes suggests that they may act as Trojan horses during early infection. Neutrophils may directly kill parasites through the diverse arsenal of antimicrobial effector mechanisms these cells possess. Through release of tissue destructive metalloproteinases and uncontrolled release of proinflammatory cytokines, PMN may contribute to immunopathology that often accompanies infection.

Mice depleted of neutrophils with a Ly6C/G-specific monoclonal antibody display increased susceptibility to infection, decreased proinflammatory cytokine responses and defective dendritic cell responses [15, 55, 60, 61]. This suggests that neutrophils are involved in protection and promotion of immunity *in vivo*. However, while the depletion result was originally interpreted to indicate a protective role for PMN, more recent studies have suggested this may not be the case. The ambiguity comes from the fact that the Ly6C/G determinant (also called Gr-1) is now known to lack complete neutrophil specificity. In addition to being expressed at high level on PMN, Gr-1 is found on certain DC subsets and on inflammatory monocytes [62]. Indeed, a recent study using a Ly6G-reactive antibody with increased specificity for neutrophils provided evidence that these cells were not required for resistance, although it was suggested that they are involved in pathology [63].

Regardless of this ambiguity, there is little doubt that PMN are active participants during the *in vivo* response to infection. Two-photon scanning-laser microscopy has been used to follow migration of PMN in draining lymph nodes of mice infected by injection into the ear flap [64]. These studies revealed that neutrophils enter the lymph node shortly after infection in a manner dependent upon MyD88, and that a significant number harbor intact parasites. Most interestingly, neutrophils displayed a previously unrecognized "swarming" behavior in the lymph node that was coordinated in space and time with egress of parasites from infected cells. Swarming of neutrophils was also associated with removal of CD169$^+$ subcapsular macrophages, possibly as a result of matrix metalloproteinase release. The ability of neutrophils to form large swarms near sites of parasites reinforces the concept that locally high numbers of these cells can significantly impact infection with *Toxoplasma* either through release of microbicidal molecules or through release of immunoregulatory cytokines and chemokines. It also seems possible that neutrophil swarming to freshly egressed parasites would favor their preferential infection.

We employed an i. p. infection model to examine the role of CXCR2 during *Toxoplasma* infection. The CXCR2 chemokine receptor recognizes IL-8-like chemokines in mice that are involved in PMN recruitment. As expected, infection of CXCR2$^{-/-}$ mice resulted in impaired neutrophil recruitment to the peritoneal cavity associated with increased parasite number at the site of infection, as well as increased cyst establishment during chronic infection [65]. While IL-12 levels did not differ between wild-type and knockout mouse strains, the amount of IFN-γ following infection was lower in the absence of CXCR2. These results clearly argue for a protective role of PMN during i. p. *T. gondii* infection, and we are currently examining responses of CXCR2$^{-/-}$ mice after orally initiated infection.

Recruitment of large numbers of neutrophils into the intestinal mucosa is a characteristic of acute infection following oral inoculation of *Toxoplasma*. Thus, within 4 days of infection, increased numbers of neutrophils are found in the lamina propria and mesenteric lymph nodes [28]. This early recruitment is dependent upon MyD88 signaling, and MyD88-dependent PMN recruitment is also observed in the peritoneal cavity following i. p. injection of parasites. Similarly, neutrophil recruitment during other infections including *Citrobacter rodentium* and *Chlamydia pneumoniae* is also dependent upon MyD88 signaling [66, 67]. A likely scenario is that TLR signaling through MyD88 at sites of infection leads to production of IL-8-like chemokines that are potent PMN chemoattractants. Possibly in addition to this, it has been reported that *Toxoplasma* itself produces factors that are directly chemotactic for neutrophils [68].

Recently, IL-17/IL-17 receptor mediated signaling has emerged as an important component of neutrophil granulopoiesis in the bone marrow and recruitment to peripheral tissues [69, 70]. Two independent studies confirmed that neutrophil numbers were lower in the ileum following infection of IL-17 receptor knockout mice [71, 72]. In both cases this was associated with decreased inflammation and pathology in the intestine. Nevertheless, for reasons that are unclear, one study found that lack of IL-17/IL-17 receptor signaling lead to increased susceptibility while the other found an increase in resistance to *T. gondii* infection.

It has become apparent that gut flora is an important player in the host-pathogen interaction during oral infection with *Toxoplasma*. Infection at doses causing proinflammatory pathology is associated with a change in the gut flora from gram-positive to overwhelmingly gram-negative species, as well as bacterial translocation into the intestinal mucosa [23, 73]. Based on studies in mice depleted of gut flora by antibiotic treatment, it was concluded that endogenous bacteria play a role in the pathology triggered by *Toxoplasma* [24]. Ileitis in this model was also found to be mediated by TLR4-dependent sensing of intestinal bacteria. Another recent report provided evidence that under lower dose parasite infection, endogenous flora provide a TLR-dependent adjuvant effect in triggering parasite-specific adaptive immunity [25]. Therefore, it is possible that neutrophil recruitment during oral infection is driven by host exposure to translocating bacteria that are known to be potent activators and recruiters of PMN, rather than being a direct response to *Toxoplasma* – or, perhaps more likely, the response may be driven by the combined activities of gut flora and the parasite itself.

CONCLUSIONS AND FUTURE DIRECTIONS

Neutrophils are an often overlooked cell type that are dismissed as primitive cells that provide temporary defense until more sophisticated immune cells such as dendritic cells, macrophages and lymphocytes respond to infection. Yet, it is clear that the neutrophil is a multi-faceted cell and there remains much to learn about the roles this fascinating cell play during the immune response [74]. The capacity of these cells to make immunoregulatory cytokines, their ability to produce extracellular DNA traps, and their unique swarming behavior in the lymph node are each examples of neutrophil functions that have previously gone unrecognized. For *Toxoplasma,* the challenge for the future is to determine the *in vivo* role of these cells during infection (Fig. **2**). Under what conditions are they harmful? When are they protective? What are the ways they mediate host protection? Finding the answers to these questions will be an important challenge for the future.

ACKNOWLEDGEMENTS

Our work on neutrophils was supported by NIH grant AI47888.

REFERENCES

[1]   Dubey JP. The history and life-cycle of *Toxoplasma gondii*. In: Weiss LM, Kim K, Eds. Toxoplasma gondii The model apicomplexan: Perspective and methods. San Diego: Academic Press 2007; 1-17.

[2]   Montoya JG, Liesenfeld O. Toxoplasmosis. Lancet 2004;363:1965-76.

[3]   Pfaff AW, Liesenfeld O, Candolfi E. Congenital toxoplasmosis. In: Ajioka JW, Soldati D, Eds. *Toxoplasma* molecular and cellular biology. Norfolk: Horizon Bioscienc; 2007; 93-110.

[4]   Sibley LD. *Toxoplasma gondii*: perfecting an intracellular life style. Traffic 2003;4:581-58.

[5]   Courret N, Darche S, Sonigo P, Milon G, Buzoni-Gatel D, Tardieux I. CD11c and CD11b expressing mouse leukocytes transport single *Toxoplasma gondii* tachyzoites to the brain. Blood 2006;107:309-16.

[6]   Gazzinelli R, Xu Y, Hieny S, Cheever A, Sher A. Simultaneous depletion of CD4$^+$ and CD8$^+$ T lymphocytes is required to reactivate chronic infection with *Toxoplasma gondii*. J Immunol 1992;149:175-80.

[7]   Luft BJ, Remington JS. Toxoplasmic encephalitis in AIDS. Clin Infect Dis 1992;15:211-22.

[8]   Suzuki Y, Conley FK, Remington JS. Importance of endogenous IFN-γ for the prevention of toxoplasmic encephalitis in mice. J Immunol 1989;143:2045-50.

[9]   Denkers EY, Gazzinelli RT. Regulation and function of T cell-mediated immunity during *Toxoplasma gondii* infection. Clin Microbiol Rev 1998;11:569-88.

[10]   Gazzinelli RT, Wysocka M, Hayashi S, *et al.* Parasite-induced IL-12 stimulates early IFN-γ synthesis and resistance during acute infection with *Toxoplasma gondii*. J Immunol 1994;153:2533-43.

[11]   Scharton-Kersten TM, Wynn TA, Denkers EY, *et al.* In the absence of endogenous IFN-γ, mice develop unimpaired IL-12 responses to Toxoplasma gondii while failing to control acute infection. J Immunol 1996;157:4045-54.

[12]   Yap G, Pesin M, Sher A. IL-12 is required for the maintenance of IFN-γ production in T cells mediating chronic resistance to the intracellular pathogen, *Toxoplasma gondii*. J Immunol 2000;165:628-31.

[13]   Denkers EY, Yap G, Scharton-Kersten T, *et al.* Perforin-mediated cytolysis plays a limited role in host resistance to *Toxoplasma gondii*. J Immunol 1997;159:1903-8.

[14]   Gazzinelli RT, Hakim FT, Hieny S, Shearer GM, Sher A. Synergistic role of CD4$^+$ and CD8$^+$ T lymphocytes in IFN-γ production and protective immunity induced by an attenuated *T. gondii* vaccine. J Immunol 1991;146:286-92.

[15]   Scharton-Kersten T, Yap G, Magram J, Sher A. Inducible nitric oxide is essential for host control of persistent but not acute infection with the intracellular pathogen *Toxoplasma gondii*. J Exp Med 1997;185:1-13.

[16]   Zhao YO, Rohde C, Lilue JT, *et al.* Toxoplasma gondii and the Immunity-Related GTPase (IRG) resistance system in mice: a review. Mem Inst Oswaldo Cruz 2009;104:234-40.

[17]   Gazzinelli RT, Wysocka M, Hieny S, *et al.* In the absence of endogenous IL-10, mice acutely infected with *Toxoplasma gondii* succumb to a lethal immune response dependent upon CD4$^+$ T cells and accompanied by overproduction of IL-12, IFN-γ, and TNF-α. J Immunol 1996;157:798-805.

[18]   Wilson EH, Wille-Reece U, Dzierszinski F, Hunter CA. A critical role for IL-10 in limiting inflammation during toxoplasmic encephalitis. J Neuroimmunol 2005;165:63-74.

[19]   Suzuki Y, Sher A, Yap G, *et al.* IL-10 is required for prevention of necrosis in the small intestine and mortality in both genetically resistant BALB/c and susceptible C57BL/6 mice following peroral infection with *Toxoplasma gondii*. J Immunol 2000;164:5375-82.

[20]   Gavrilescu LC, Denkers EY. IFN-γ overproduction and high level apoptosis are associated with high but not low virulence *Toxoplasma gondii* infection. J Immunol 2001;167:902-9.

[21]   Mordue DG, Monroy F, La Regina M, Dinarello CA, Sibley LD. Acute toxoplasmosis leads to lethal overproduction of Th1 cytokines. J Immunol 2001;167:4574-84.

[22]   Liesenfeld O, Kosek J, Remington JS, Suzuki Y. Association of CD4$^+$ T cell-dependent, IFN-γ-mediated necrosis of the small intestine with genetic susceptibility of mice to peroral infection with *Toxoplasma gondii*. J Exp Med 1996;184:597-607.

[23]   Heimesaat MM, Bereswill S, Fischer A, *et al.* Gram-Negative Bacteria Aggravate Murine Small Intestinal Th1-Type Immunopathology following Oral Infection with Toxoplasma gondii. J Immunol 2006;177:8785-95.

[24]   Heimesaat MM, Fischer A, Jahn HK, *et al.* Exacerbation of Murine Ileitis By Toll-Like Receptor 4 Meditated Sensing of Lipopolysaccharide From Commensal Escherichia coli. Gut 2007;56:941-8.

[25]   Benson A, Pifer R, Behrendt CL, Hooper LV, Yarovinsky F. Gut commensal bacteria direct a protective immune response against Toxoplasma gondii. Cell Host Microbe 2009;6:187-96.

[26]   Denkers EY. Toll-like receptor initiated host defense against Toxoplasma gondii. J Biomed Biotechnol 2010;2010:737125.

[27]   Scanga CA, Aliberti J, Jankovic D, *et al*. Cutting edge: MyD88 is required for resistance to *Toxoplasma gondii* infection and regulates parasite-induced IL-12 production by dendritic cells. J Immunol 2002;168:5997-6001.

[28]   Sukhumavasi W, Egan CE, Warren AL, *et al*. TLR adaptor MyD88 is essential for pathogen control during oral toxoplasma gondii infection but not adaptive immunity induced by a vaccine strain of the parasite. J Immunol 2008;181:3464-73.

[29]   Plattner F, Yarovinsky F, Romero S, *et al*. Toxoplasma profilin is essential for host cell invasion and TLR dependent induction of interleukin-12. Cell Host and Microbe 2008;14:77-87.

[30]   Yarovinsky F, Zhang D, Anderson JF, *et al*. TLR11 activation of dendritic cells by a protozoan profilin-like protein. Science 2005;308:1626-9.

[31]   Debierre-Grockiego F, Campos MA, Azzouz N, *et al*. Activation of TLR2 and TLR4 by glycosylphosphatidylinositols derived from Toxoplasma gondii. J Immunol 2007;179:1129-37.

[32]   Foureau DM, Mielcarz DW, Menard LC, *et al*. TLR9-dependent induction of intestinal alpha-defensins by Toxoplasma gondii. J Immunol 2010;184:7022-9.

[33]   Minns LA, Menard LC, Foureau DM, *et al*. TLR9 Is Required for the Gut-Associated Lymphoid Tissue Response following Oral Infection of Toxoplasma gondii. J Immunol 2006;176:7589-97.

[34]   Bierly AL, Shufesky WJ, Sukhumavasi W, Morelli A, Denkers EY. Dendritic cells expressing plasmacytoid marker PDCA-1 are Trojan horses during Toxoplasma gondii infection. J Immunol 2008;181:8445-91.

[35]   Liu CH, Fan YT, Dias A, *et al*. Cutting Edge: Dendritic Cells Are Essential for *In Vivo* IL-12 Production and Development of Resistance against Toxoplasma gondii Infection in Mice. J Immunol 2006;177:31-5.

[36]   Lambert H, Vutova PP, Adams WC, Lore K, Barragan A. The Toxoplasma gondii-Shuttling Function of Dendritic Cells is Linked to the Parasite Genotype. Infect Immun 2009.

[37]   Dunay IR, Damatta RA, Fux B, *et al*. Gr1(+) Inflammatory Monocytes Are Required for Mucosal Resistance to the Pathogen Toxoplasma gondii. Immunity 2008;29:306-17.

[38]   Lykens JE, Terrell CE, Zoller EE, *et al*. Mice with a selective impairment of IFN-γ signaling in macrophage lineage cells demonstrate the critical role of IFN-γ-activated macrophages for the control of protozoan parasitic infections *in vivo*. J Immunol 2010;184:877-85.

[39]   Erbe DV, Pfefferkorn ER, Fanger MW. Functions of the various IgG Fc receptors in mediating killing of Toxoplasma gondii. J Immunol 1991;146:3145-51.

[40]   Nakao M, Konishi E. Proliferation of *Toxoplasma gondii* in human neutrophils *in vitro*. Parasitol 1991;103:23-7.

[41]   Wilson CB, Remington JS. Activity of human blood leukocytes against *Toxoplasma gondii*. J Infect Dis 1979;140:890-5.

[42]   Channon JY, Miselis KA, Minns LA, Dutta C, Kasper LH. *Toxoplasma gondii* induces granulocyte colony-stimulating factor and granulocyte-macrophage colony-stimulating factor secretion by human fibroblasts: implications for neutrophil apoptosis. Infect Immun 2002;70:6048-57.

[43]   Cassatella MA. Neutrophil-derived proteins: Selling cytokines by the pound. Adv Immunol 1999;73:369-509.

[44]   Lloyd AR, Oppenheim JJ. Poly's lament: the neglected role of the polymorphonuclear neutrophil in the afferent limb of the immune response. Immunol Today 1992;13:169-72.

[45]   Denkers EY, Del Rio L, Bennouna S. Neutrophil production of IL-12 and other cytokines during microbial infection. Chem Immunol Allergy 2003;83:95-114.

[46]   Bliss SK, Marshall AJ, Zhang Y, Denkers EY. Human polymorphonuclear leukocytes produce IL-12, TNF-α, and the chemokines macrophage-inflammatory protein-1α and -1☐ in response to *Toxoplasma gondii* antigens. J Immunol 1999;162:7369-75.

[47]   Bliss SK, Zhang Y, Denkers EY. Murine neutrophil stimulation by *Toxoplasma gondii* antigen drives high level production of IFN-γ-independent IL-12. J Immunol 1999;163:2081-8.

[48]   Bliss SK, Butcher BA, Denkers EY. Rapid recruitment of neutrophils with prestored IL-12 during microbial infection. J Immunol 2000;165:4515-21.

[49]   Brandt E, Woerly G, Ben Younes A, Loiseau S, Capron M. IL-4 production by human polymorphonuclear neutrophils. J Leukoc Biol 2000;68:125-30.

[50]   Matzer SP, Baumann T, Lukacs NW, Rollinghoff M, Beuscher HU. Constitutive expression of macrophage-inflammatory protein 2 (MIP-2) mRNA in bone marrow gives rise to peripheral neutrophils with preformed MIP-2 protein. J Immunol 2001;167:4635-43.

[51]   Terebuh PD, Otterness IG, Strieter RM, *et al*. Biologic and immunohistochemical analysis of interleukin-6 expression *in vivo*. Constitutive and induced expression in murine polymorphonuclear and mononuclear phagocytes. Am J Pathol 1992;140:649-57.

[52] Del Rio L, Butcher BA, Bennouna S, Hieny S, Sher A, Denkers EY. *Toxoplasma gondii* triggers MyD88-dependent and CCL2(MCP-1) responses using distinct parasite molecules and host receptors. J Immunol 2004;172:6954-60.

[53] Sukhumavasi W, Egan CE, Denkers EY. Mouse neutrophils require JNK2 MAPK for Toxoplasma gondii-induced IL-12p40 and CCL2/MCP-1 release. J Immunol 2007;179:3570-7.

[54] Denkers EY, Butcher BA, Del Rio L, Bennouna S. Neutrophils, dendritic cells and *Toxoplasma*. Internat J Parasitol 2004;34:411-21.

[55] Bennouna S, Bliss SK, Curiel TJ, Denkers EY. Cross-talk in the innate immune system: neutrophils instruct early recruitment and activation of dendritic cells during microbial infection. J Immunol 2003;171:6052-8.

[56] van Gisbergen KP, Ludwig IS, Geijtenbeek TB, van Kooyk Y. Interactions of DC-SIGN with Mac-1 and CEACAM1 regulate contact between dendritic cells and neutrophils. FEBS Lett 2005;579:6159-68.

[57] van Gisbergen KP, Sanchez-Hernandez M, Geijteenbeek TB, van Kooyk Y. Neutrophils mediate immune modulation of dendritic cells through glycosylation-dependent interactions between Mac-1 and DC-SIGN. J Exp Med 2005;201:1281-92.

[58] van Gisbergen KP, Geijtenbeek TB, van Kooyk Y. Close encounters of neutrophils and DCs. Trends Immunol 2005;26:626-31.

[59] Charmoy M, Brunner-Agten S, Aebischer D, et al. Neutrophil-derived CCL3 is essential for the rapid recruitment of dendritic cells to the site of Leishmania major inoculation in resistant mice. PLoS Pathog 2010;6:e1000755.

[60] Bliss SK, Gavrilescu LC, Alcaraz A, Denkers EY. Neutrophil depletion during *Toxoplasma gondii* infection leads to impaired immunity and lethal systemic pathology. Infect Immun 2001;69:4898-905.

[61] Sayles PC, Johnson LJ. Exacerbation of toxoplasmosis in neutrophil depleted mice. Nat Immun 1997;15:249-58.

[62] Egan CE, Sukhumavasi W, Bierly AL, Denkers EY. Understanding the multiple functions of Gr-1[+] cell subpopulations during microbial infection. Immunologic Res 2008;40:35-48.

[63] Dunay IR, Fuchs A, Sibley LD. Inflammatory monocytes but not neutrophils are necessary to control infection with Toxoplasma gondii in mice. Infect Immun 2010;78:1564-70.

[64] Chtanova T, Schaeffer M, Han SJ, et al. Dynamics of Neutrophil Migration in Lymph Nodes during Infection. Immunity 2008;29:487-96.

[65] Del Rio L, Bennouna S, Salinas J, Denkers EY. CXCR2 deficiency confers impaired neutrophil recruitment and increased susceptibility during *Toxoplasma gondii* infection. J Immunol 2001;167:6503-9.

[66] Lebeis SL, Bommarius B, Parkos CA, Sherman MA, Kalman D. TLR signaling mediated by MyD88 is required for a protective innate immune response by neutrophils to Citrobacter rodentium. J Immunol 2007;179:566-77.

[67] Rodriguez N, Fend F, Jennen L, et al. Polymorphonuclear neutrophils improve replication of Chlamydia pneumoniae *in vivo* upon MyD88-dependent attraction. J Immunol 2005;174:4836-44.

[68] Nakao M, Konishi E. Neutrophil chemotactic factors secreted from *Toxoplasma gondii*. Parasitol 1991;103:29-34.

[69] Miyamoto M, Prause O, Sjostrand M, Laan M, Lotvall J, Linden A. Endogenous IL-17 as a mediator of neutrophil recruitment caused by endotoxin exposure in mouse airways. J Immunol 2003;170:4665-72.

[70] Ye P, Rodriguez FH, Kanaly S, et al. Requirement of interleukin 17 receptor signaling for lung CXC chemokine and granulocyte colony-stimulating factor expression, neutrophil recruitment, and host defense. J Exp Med 2001;194:519-27.

[71] Guiton R, Vasseur V, Charron S, et al. Interleukin 17 receptor signaling is deleterious during Toxoplasma gondii infection in susceptible BL6 mice. J Infect Dis 2010;202:427-35.

[72] Kelly MN, Kolls JK, Happel K, et al. Interleukin-17/interleukin-17 receptor-mediated signaling is important for generation of an optimal polymorphonuclear response against *Toxoplasma gondii* infection. Infect Immun 2005;73:617-21.

[73] Egan CE, Craven MD, Leng J, Mack M, Simpson KW, Denkers EY. CCR2-dependent intraepithelial lymphocytes mediate inflammatory gut pathology during Toxoplasma gondii infection. Mucosal Immunol 2009;2:527-35.

[74] Nathan C. Neutrophils and immunity: challenges and opportunities. Nat Rev Immunol 2006;6:173-82.

CHAPTER 8

Neutrophils as Potential Safe Niche for *Leishmania* and *Anaplasma*

Ger van Zandbergen[1,*], Elena Bank[1], Martina Behnen[2], Matthias Klinger[3] and Tamas Laskay[2]

[1]*Institute for Medical Microbiology and Hygiene, University Clinic of Ulm, Albert Einstein Allee 11, D-89081, Germany;* [2]*Institute of Medical Microbiology and Hygiene, University of Lübeck, Ratzeburger Allee 160, D-23562 Lübeck, Germany and* [3]*Institute of Anatomy, University of Lübeck, Ratzeburger Allee 160, D-23562, Germany*

Abstract: Neutrophils are the most crucial cells for early defence against infections. When properly activated they can kill extracellular pathogens but also also obligate intracellular pathogens such as *Leishmania* and *Anaplasma*. However, once the phagocytotic killing has been evaded, neutrophils can serve as host cells for obligate intracellular pathogens. Parasitized neutrophils were shown to function as a 'Trojan horse', to silently transfer *Leishmania* to macrophages as well as *Anaplasma* to other neutrophils. Here, we discuss the Trojan horse function of neutrophils for *Leishmania* and *Anaplasma*.

INTRODUCTION

Leishmaniasis is a parasitic infection with the genus *Leishmania* (family: *Trypanosomatidae*, order: *Kinetoplastida*) which affects 88 countries and threatens 350 million people in tropical and subtropical regions of the world. The causative agent of leishmaniasis is a dimorphic unicellular parasite that lives and replicates in the gut of sand flies as a flagellated promastigote form or in mammalian cells as an aflagellated amastigote form. This adaptation to both an arthropod vector and a mammalian host is a typical feature of the obligatory intracellular parasite [1]. The insect vector of *Leishmania* is the sand fly of the subgenera *Phlebotomus* and *Lutzomyia* [2]. The infection with different species of *Leishmania* causes various forms of leishmaniasis including cutaneous (CL), mucocutaneous (ML) and visceral (VL) ranging from self healing lesions to a severe organ-infiltrating disease. The basic pathogenesis of *Leishmania* infection has been deciphered using experimental mouse infection models as well as human cell-based *in vitro* experiments, reviewed by [3, 4].

To escape the host immune response after injection into the skin by a sand fly bite, the *Leishmania* parasites have evolved strategies to be internalized by host cells, hiding inside them to ensure their survival. *Leishmania* need macrophages to develop into multiplying amastigotes resulting in disease development. Inside macrophages the parasites are located within specialized compartments, called phagolysosomes, where they differentiate into non-motile amastigotes, which are adapted to the acidic and hydrolase-rich conditions within the phagolysosome and responsible for the maintenance and propagation of the infection [3]. Therefore, research has focussed on these host cells to first understand pathogenesis. For better understanding leishmaniasis, research has shifted in the last decade focussing on other potential host cells able to shape the immune response. It is now clear that *Leishmania* parasites are also detectable in human and murine dendritic cells (DCs), murine fibroblasts as well as in both human and murine neutrophils [5-7]. In this E-book chapter we focus on the role of neutrophils as potential safe niche for *Leishmania* and other neutrophil targeting pathogens like *Anaplasma phagocytophilum* (*A. phagocytophilum*). It leads to us to the conclusion that neutrophil effector functions can be silenced resulting in a suitable host for both *Leishmania* and *A. phagocytophilum*.

THE ROLE OF NEUTROPHILS IN THE IMMUNE RESPONSE

Neutrophils are classical well known phagocytes contributing to the 'first line of defence' against infectious agents or 'non-self' substances which get through the body's physical barriers [8]. Neutrophils provide an important link between the innate and adaptive immune system [6, 8, 9]. It was recently published that neutrophils can influence the recruitment of DCs to the site of infection via secretion of CCL3 [10]. Still, neutrophils are one of the most

Address correspondence to Ger van Zandbergen at: Institute for Medical Microbiology and Hygiene, University Clinic of Ulm, Albert-Einstein-Allee 11, D-89081 Ulm, Germany; E-mail: Ger.Zandbergen@uniklinik-ulm.de

underappreciated immune cells of the immune system and many neutrophil functions remain to be discovered. Neutrophils are heavily armed with an impressive array of antimicrobial arsenal but once killing is evaded by pathogens, they become host cells [11]. After a short life span neutrophils die by apoptosis leading to their phagocytosis by macrophages.

RECRUITMENT OF NEUTROPHILS

Neutrophils rapidly accumulate at the site of pathogen infection [12] but the factors involved in this recruitment are still not well defined and may include chemokines, cytokines and other molecules secreted by the parasite and/or host. Thus, there are controversial positions about the possible mechanisms for the homing of neutrophils and silent uptake of pathogens. Some authors call for a concept that tissue damage caused by needle injection or sand fly bite results in a robust infiltration of neutrophils, whereas others favour a recruitment-modulatory function of parasite and vector derived molecules [12, 13]. Most likely there is an overlapping of neutrophil migration by side effects caused by local destruction of the microvasculature after dermal inoculation with the arthropod proboscis or a needle [12].

Neutrophils are responsive to IL-8, a chemokine which is secreted by epithelial cells, keratinocytes, fibroblasts and endothelial cells but also by neutrophils themselves. Human neutrophils were shown to release IL-8 in response to *Leishmania major in vitro,* a process that should promote their own migration [14]. Thus, IL-8 may modulate the early neutrophil recruitment to the site of infection, but a direct involvement during infection *in vivo* remains to be demonstrated.

A *Leishmania* chemotactic factor (LCF) was shown to specifically recruit neutrophils to the site of infection [14] and this LCF was demonstrated to interact with the chemokine receptor Lipoxin A4 receptor (ALX) [15]. This interaction resulted in an increased silent uptake of *Leishmania* promastigotes and a higher level of intracellular survival [15]. The saliva of most blood-feeding arthropods contains vasodilators, anti-aggregation factors, and anti-coagulants that could affect the migration of potential host cells [16]. It was reported that a combination of *Leishmania* parasites and saliva from *Lutzomia longipalpis* enhances the influx of neutrophils and macrophages in susceptible BALB/c mice but not in resistant C57BL/6 mice [17]. This suggests that the attracting function of saliva depends on the genetic background of the mouse strain used for experiments.

PATHOGEN KILLING BY NEUTROPHILS

Neutrophils are equipped with various antimicrobial functions and armed with toxic oxygen radicals, lytic enzymes and cationic proteins. After entry of infectious agents the neutrophils are stimulated to phagocytose and also to secrete factors involved in the recruitment and/or activation of other inflammatory cells. The killing of pathogens is often accompanied by release of antimicrobial molecules into the extracellular milieu. Human neutrophils are shown to release granule proteins and chromatin that together form extracellular fibres (or neutrophil extracellular traps; NETs) that bind and kill pathogens (reviewed by V. Brinkmann *et al.* in this Ebook) [8]. Both mechanisms are related and play a role in the killing of microorganisms before their complete engulfment [8, 18, 19]. Recently it was demonstrated that *Leishmania* was ensnared by NETs released by human neutrophils and furthermore that its surface lipophosphoglycan induced NET-formation [20]. After phagocytosis the pathogens end up within hours in phagolysosomes by fusion with lysosomes, enriched with antimicrobial peptides, reactive oxygen species (ROS) and degrading enzymes [21]. Neutrophils are able to produce nitric oxide (NO) by iNOS and thereby kill pathogens. Concordantly, neutrophils expressing iNOS were found in lesions of C57BL/6 mice infected with *Leishmania major* and *Leishmania* parasites were demonstrated to induce the production of NO in C57BL/6 mice [22, 23]. There are other mechanisms, like degranulation of cytoplasmic storage compartments (granules) within the phagolysosome which results in the release of pre-formed proteinases or antibiotic proteins involved in degradation [24]. It was shown that neutral proteases, such as neutrophil elastases (NEs) are essential for the elimination of *Leishmania* parasites [24-26] and that NEs even activate infected macrophages to kill intracellular *Leishmania* parasites via TLR4 signalling [27]. Summarized, neutrophils are well equipped effector cells of the innate immune system, ready to kill pathogens, while the *Leishmania* parasites have evolved equally mechanisms to evade killing by neutrophils. One example is the block of the oxidative burst within the neutrophils by the parasites [7]. Other species of *Leishmania*, like *Leishmania donovani* are not found inside the lytic compartments of neutrophils [28].

CAN NEUTROPHILS BE USED AS TROJAN HORSES?

There are three functions to manipulate by the parasite to get a Trojan horse out of a neutrophil. First, the neutrophils need to be recruited to the site of infection. Second, the lethal killing mechanisms have to be deactivated, so a pathogen can survive inside the cells. And third, the neutrophils should regulate their uptake by the next host cell and thus arrange the unnoticed transfer of pathogens to their final host. The chemokine receptor ALX is one target molecule mediating the recruitment of neutrophils. The receptor responds to both anti-inflammatory lipids like lipoxin A4 and bacterial chemoattractants. Additionally it was demonstrated that neutrophils activated by lipoxin A4 via the ALX receptor have a decreased oxidative burst reaction and an increased phagocytosis of apoptotic cells [29, 30]. Interestingly it was shown that *Leishmania* use the ALX receptor to deactivate neutrophils killing mechanisms. Both pre-incubation with LCF and lipoxin A4 doubled the survival of *Leishmania* promastigotes inside neutrophils [15].

We found that *L. major* promastigotes survived inside PMN up to 42 h (Fig. **1**). Electron microscopical analysis revealed the intracellular presence of intact promastigotes after 42 h of incubation in PMN. The four intracellular promastigotes show a perfectly intact body structure with a nucleus (N), a kinetoplast (K), a flagellum (F) and a flagellum pocket (FP). In addition, the nucleus (Nu) of the infected PMN is condensed as an indication that the PMN is undergoing apoptosis (Fig. **1**).

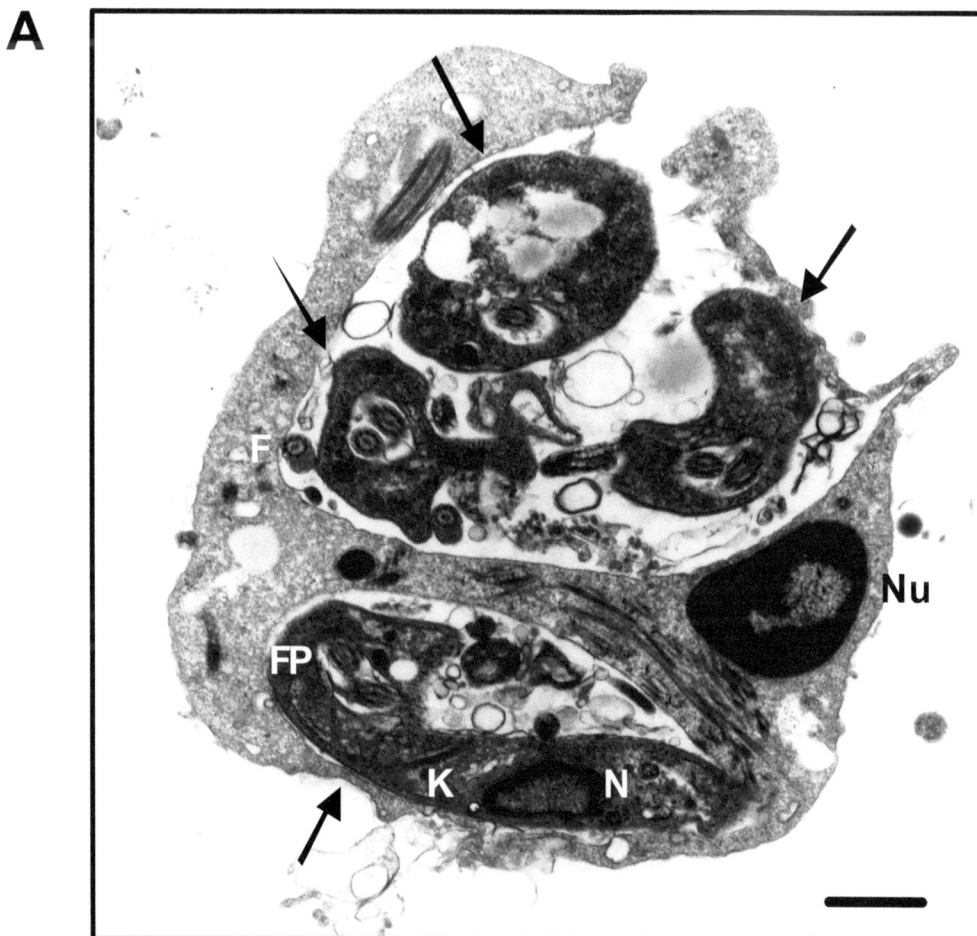

Figure 1: *L. major* promastigote-infected PMN.

Transmission electron micrograph of a PMN 42 h after infection with *L. major* promastigotes. Arrows indicate viable intracellular *Leishmania* parasites. Nucleus (Nu), kinetoplast (K), flagellum (F) and the flagellum pocket (FP) structures appear intact. A typical 9:2 structure can be observed in the flagellum and flagellum pocket sections (bar = 1 μM, magnification x10,000).

Another way to deactivate the killing mechanisms of professional phagocytes like neutrophils and macrophages is the engulfment of apoptotic cells [31]. Phosphatidylserine (PS) is an apoptotic kind of "eat me"-signal for phagocytes and induces the secretion of anti-inflammatory TGF-ß after the uptake of PS-positive cells. Dying PS-positive cells are no danger for the organism and their uptake does not induce the antimicrobial killing functions [32, 33]. *Leishmania* parasites exploit this mechanism to silence the host cell, by the virulent inoculum consisting of both viable and dying PS-positive promastigotes [34]. Successful PMN invasion depends on the expression of the "eat me" signal PS on a sub-population of apoptotic parasites. After depleting the apoptotic parasites from a virulent population, *L. major* do not survive in phagocytes *in vitro* and lose their disease inducing ability *in vivo* [34, 35]. It was shown that promastigote survival depended on the PMN production of a "forget me" signal. PMN interaction with PS positive promastigotes induced the production of TGF-ß down regulating inflammatory TNF. Moreover interaction with viable promastigotes alone induced a TNF-dependent killing of intracellular promastigotes [34, 35].

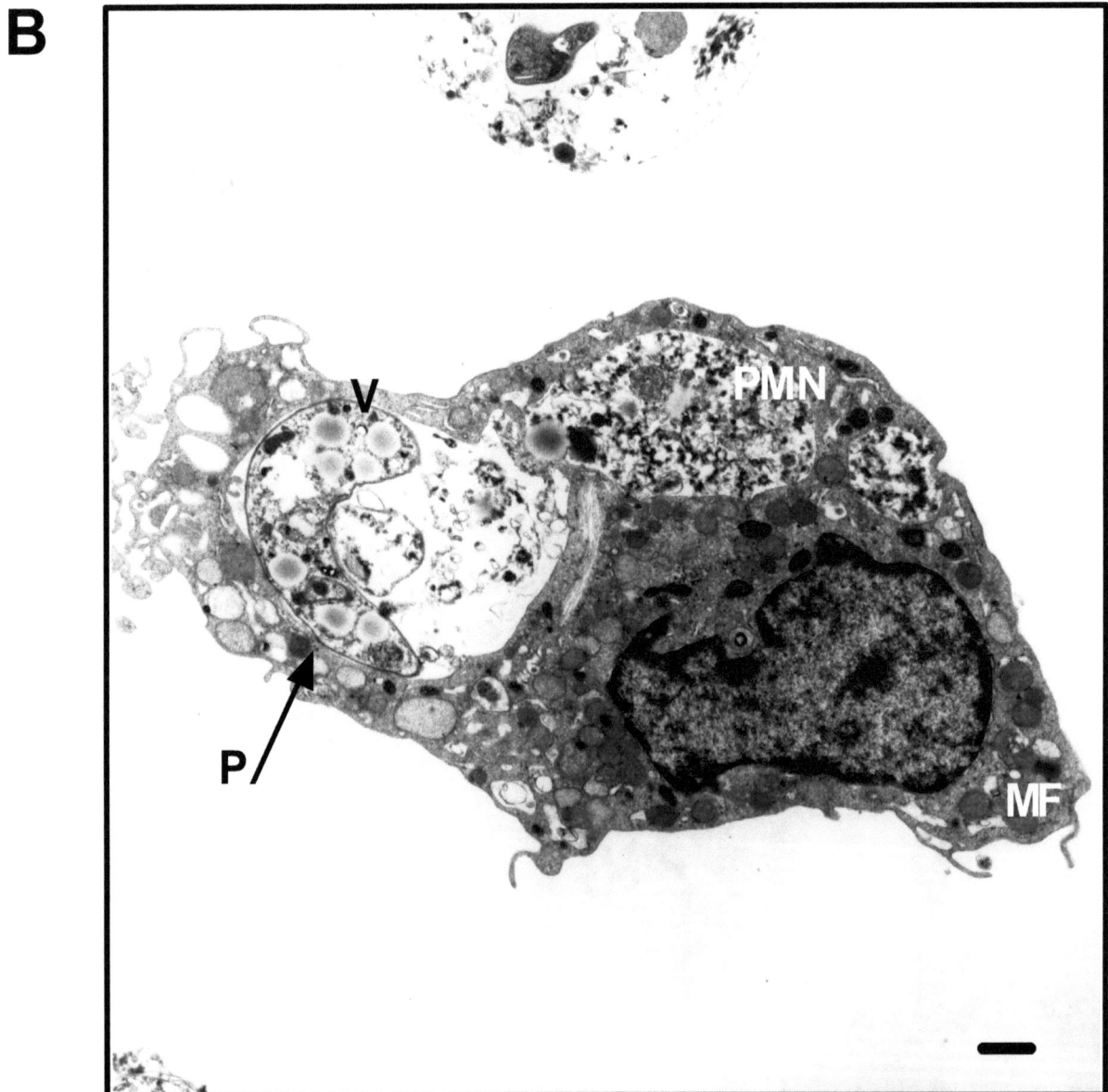

Figure 2: *L. major* promastigote transfer from infected PMN to MF.

Transmission electron micrograph of a MF 1 h after co-incubation with infected PMN. Arrow indicates a released *Leishmania* parasite (P) and the nearly digested PMN (PMN). Inside the parasite are several vacuoles (V) (bar = 1 µM, magnification x 4,500).

Uninfected neutrophils have a short lifespan and become rapidly apoptotic, but infected neutrophils with *Leishmania* are demonstrated to live longer. The apoptotic death program is delayed for up to two days, inhibiting the processing of procaspases in the infected cells [36]. In addition, infected neutrophils were shown to secrete the chemokine MIP-1b (CCL4) and recruit macrophages that way. In an experimental murine model of subcutaneous leishmaniasis it was published that the peak influx of macrophages to the site of infection coincides with the time point when infected neutrophils become PS-positive and release MIP-1b (CCL4) [37]. This suggests that recruited macrophages would meet apoptotic neutrophils hiding *Leishmania* parasites inside rather than extracellular promastigotes in the infected tissue.

The final step in converting a neutrophil into a Trojan horse is taking advantage of the fact that aging neutrophils die by apoptosis and simultaneously recruit macrophages for their uptake. For this reason the apoptotic neutrophils control their silent clearance by macrophages and thus can serve as Trojan horses. In this way infected neutrophils arrange the unnoticed transfer of parasites into their final host cells where the first stage of differentiation into amastigotes and then replication of amastigotes starts. We found that 42 h old infected PMN were ingested by human MF (Fig. **2**). The electron microscopical analysis shows that the PMN structures have disappeared and only a remaining intracellular parasite in the promastigote form is present. The many vacuoles (V) inside the parasite are suggestive for an autophagic process, taking place during stage differentiation into the amastigote stage. At the same time apoptotic PMN remains have disappeared (Fig. **2**).

In another study it was observed that *Leishmania*-containing neutrophils were not phagocytosed by macrophages, but rather *Leishmania* parasites escape neutrophils and subsequently infected macrophages [12]. Recently the arrival of recruited macrophages to the site of infection was shown to induce apoptosis of neutrophils, intensified by the presence of *Leishmania* parasites [38]. Here the apoptotic neutrophils without being infected have the function to silence the phagocytosing macrophages promoting intracellular *Leishmania* survival.

CAN NEUTROPHILS PHAGOCYTOSE OTHER APOPTOTIC CELLS?

To silence the antimicrobial mechanisms of neutrophils, apoptotic *Leishmania* parasites induce the production of the anti-inflammatory cytokine TGFβ but not the pro-inflammatory TNF in cultures of human neutrophils [34]. But until recently it was unclear whether this effect was unique for apoptotic *Leishmania* parasites or if a similar mechanism applies for other types of apoptotic cells too. However, apoptotic cells are generally well known to reduce pro-inflammatory cytokines and simultaneously induce anti-inflammatory cytokines in macrophages, which are the major phagocyte population to clear apoptotic cells [39-43]. Until recently it was not clear which effects apoptotic cells exert on the function of neutrophil granulocytes. It was not even known whether neutrophils can recognize and ingest apoptotic cells. Recently we demonstrated for the first time that neutrophils are also able to recognize and phagocytose apoptotic cells (Fig. **3**). Ingested apoptotic material is contained in acidified phagolysosomes inside neutrophils (Fig. **3**).

Importantly, the uptake of apoptotic cells/material did not result in the activation of the antimicrobial functions. Moreover, the pro-inflammatory neutrophil functions were clearly down-regulated by apoptotic cells [44]. One of the most effective microbicidal functions, the formation of an oxidative burst, is reduced by apoptotic cells. Additionally the production of pro-inflammatory cytokines by neutrophils such as TNF and IP-10 is decreased by the presence of apoptotic cells.

Both apoptotic human cells and apoptotic *Leishmania* express to some extent the same surface markers such as PS. This marker is likely to be involved in the phagocytosis process of apoptotic *Leishmania* parasites by neutrophils [34]. Moreover, similar mechanisms are likely to play a role in deactivating the neutrophil effector mechanisms, including oxidative bursts and pro-inflammatory cytokines, by apoptotic cells and thus contribute to disease development during pathogenesis of *Leishmania*. This suggests that *Leishmania* parasites exploit the physiological mechanisms of the host to avoid an unmeant inflammatory response after clearance of apoptotic cells. It was shown that virulent inoculums of *Leishmania* promastigotes consist of viable and apoptotic parasites accumulating in the stationary growth phase both *in vitro* and in sand flies [34]. The viable promastigotes alone are not able to induce a productive disease, which means that the apoptotic parasites are essential to mediate the inhibition of the antimicrobial functions of the neutrophils. There is no evidence for apoptotic mimicry or other mechanisms of *L. major* parasites to enter the host phagocytes silently.

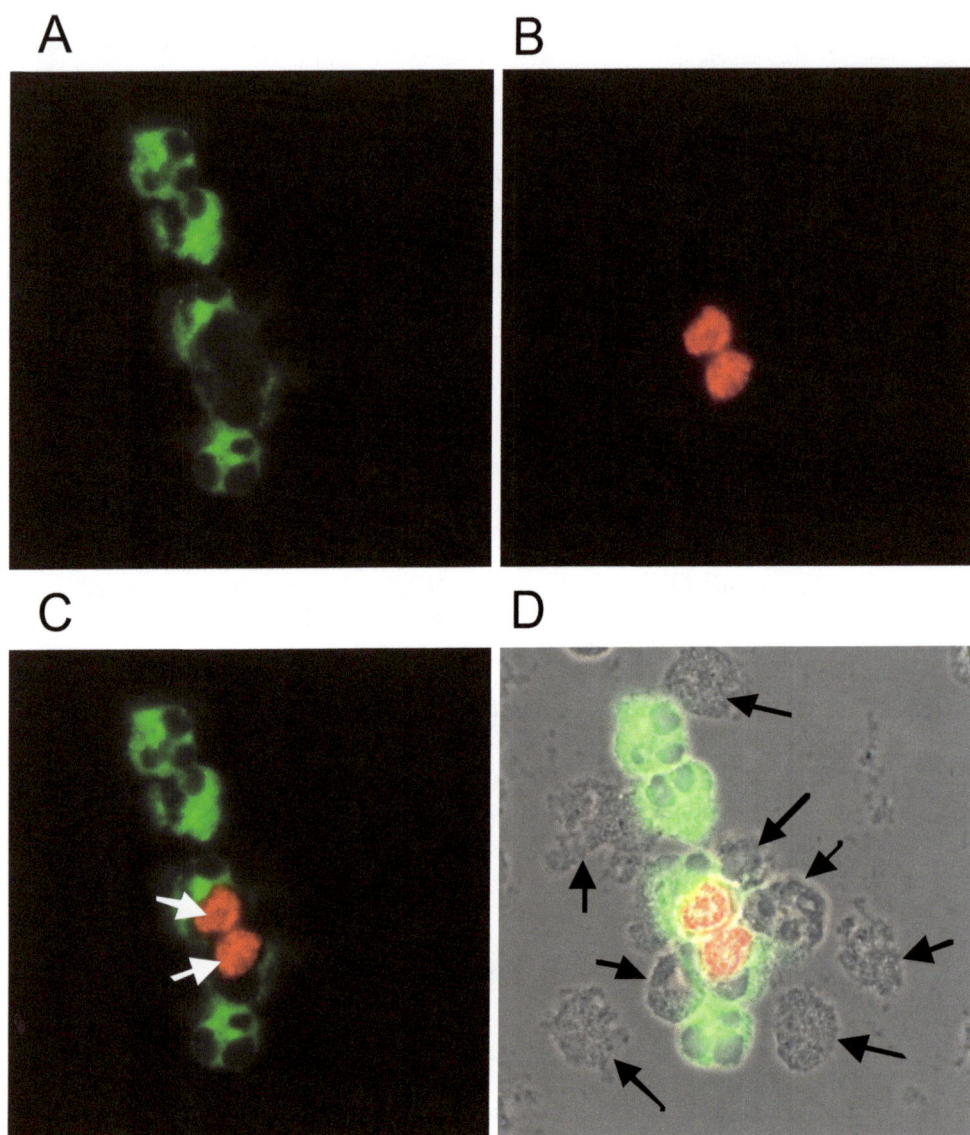

Figure 3: Neutrophils phagocytose apoptotic neutrophils. Ingested apoptotic material is contained in acidified phagolysosomes inside neutrophils. Uptake of a pHrodo-SE–labelled apoptotic neutrophil by a neutrophil granulocyte. PKH-67 (green)–labelled freshly isolated neutrophils were co-incubated for 90 min with pHrodo-SE–labelled apoptotic neutrophils in culture medium containing 30% fresh human serum and 100 ng/ml LPS;. pHrodo-SE is a pH sensitive dye which emits red fluorescent light at an increased intensity with decreasing environmental pH. In a pH neutral environment, the light emission is almost undetectable meaning that the non-phagocytosed apoptotic cells are not fluorescent or very dim. The signal, however, becomes intensive after phagocytosis and phagosome-lysosome fusion. A) green PKH-67 fluorescence, (B) red fluorescence (excitation 546 nm, emission detected through a 590-nm longpass filter), (C) overlay of green and red fluorescence, (D) overlay of green and red fluorescence with the bright field images. The red color of the cell inside of a fresh neutrophil (white arrows) indicates that the pHrodo-SE–labelled apoptotic neutrophil is located in an acidified environment inside neutrophils. Non-ingested pHrodo-SE–labelled apoptotic neutrophils are non-fluorescent (black arrows).

ANAPLASMA AND *LEISHMANIA* INFECTION: COMMON PATHWAYS OF SURVIVAL IN NEUTROPHILS

Among several pathogenic microorganisms that survive in neutrophils [11] *Anaplasma phagocytophilum* (*A. phagocytophilum*) is the only one specialized for neutrophils. *A. phagocytophilum* is a tick-borne obligate intracellular Gram-negative bacterium that infects neutrophil granulocytes of mammals, including man [45]. The niche for *A. phagocytophilum*, the neutrophil, indicates that the pathogen has developed adaptations and pathogenic mechanisms suggesting that *Anaplasma* actively subverts innate immune responses. Inside host neutrophils, *A. phagocytophilum* survives in cytoplasmic vacuoles and inhibits their fusion with lysosomes [46]. The bacteria replicate within the host cell vacuole forming a microcolony called a morula [47, 48]. As additional escape mechanisms, the bacteria inhibit the production of reactive oxygen species [49-51], delay PMN apoptosis, and exploit the neutrophil chemokine response (reviewed in [11, 52]). Since *A. phagocytophilum* completes its life cycle in neutrophils, all these escape mechanisms appear to be crucial to subvert the antimicrobial effector machinery of neutrophils and make them suitable niche for microbial survival and growth. A more recent study from our laboratory revealed invaluable details how *Anaplasma* can prevent neutrophil activation [53]. It was shown that IFNγ signalling, which is supposed to result in activation of neutrophil effector functions [54], is compromised in *Anaplasma*-infected cells [53]. A markedly decreased expression of the IFNγ receptor on the surface of *A. phagocytophilum*-infected PMN was observed as well as a diminished IFNγ-induced STAT1 phosphorylation. Importantly, a strong upregulation of the negative regulators SOCS1 and SOCS3 was observed in infected cells. As a consequence of compromised IFNγ-signalling, *A. phagocytophilum*-infection led to a markedly reduced secretion of IFNγ-inducible chemokines IP-10/CXCL10 and MIG/CXCL9. These data show that *A. phagocytophilum*-infection leads to compromised IFNγ-signalling in infected neutrophils. Since IP-10/CXCL10 secretion was reported to be downregulated in neutrophils after infection with *L. major* ([14], *Leishmania*-infection, similarly to *Anaplasma*, is likely to inhibit IFNγ-signalling in neutrophils. As generally accepted, the Th1 cytokine IFNγ provides a crucial activating stimulus for macrophages infected with intracellular pathogens among others *Mycobacteria* and *Leishmania*. It is, therefore, quite conceivable that intracellular pathogens evolved mechanisms that interfere with IFNγ-signalling in macrophages [55-57]. The above mentioned studies with neutrophils infected with *Anaplasma* [53] and *Leishmania* [14] suggest that similar mechanisms apply for macrophages and neutrophils. It means that intracellular pathogens target IFNγ-signalling not only in macrophages but in neutrophils as well. Available data strongly suggest that inhibition of IFNγ-signalling contributes to the survival of *Leishmania* parasites in neutrophils.

MATERIAL AND METHODS

Culture of *Leishmania major* Promastigotes and Generation of Neutrophil Granulocytes and Macrophages

Stationary phase *L. major* (MHOM/IL/81/FEBNI) promastigotes were collected from *in vitro* cultures in biphasic NNN blood agar medium as described by [29]. Neutrophil granulocytes (PMN) and monocytes were isolated from buffy coat blood from healthy adult volunteers as previously described [29]. The purity of granulocytes was always > 99 % as determined microscopically after Giemsa staining of cytocentrifuge slides (Thermo Shandon, Pittsburgh, PA). The viability of cells was > 99 % as assessed by trypan blue dye exclusion. Macrophages (MF) were generated by culturing autologous monocytes for 2 days in complete RPMI 1640 medium supplemented with 10 ng/ml M-CSF (Peprotech).

Infection of Human PMN and MF with *L. Major* Promastigotes

PMN (1×10^7/ml) were isolated and co-incubated with *L. major* promastigotes at 37°C and 5 % CO^2 at a parasite to PMN ratio of 5:1 in complete RPMI 1640 medium (Invitrogen Life Technologies, Grand Island, NY), supplemented with 10 % heat inactivated FCS, 50 μM 2-Mercaptoethanol, 2 mM L-glutamine, 10 mM HEPES, 100 μg/ml penicillin, and 160 μg/ml gentamicin, all obtained from Seromed-Biochrom (Berlin, Germany) [23]. Extracellular parasites were removed after 3 h of co-incubation (for phagocytosis experiments with parasitized PMN and MF). After 42 h of infection this procedure yielded a population of infected PMN in which the ratio of extracellular *L. major* promastigotes was < 1 per 1000 PMN. Infection rates and number of parasites per PMN were determined by microscopical counting of at least 200 Giemsa stained cells. Subsequently infected PMN were co-incubated with MF at a parasite to macrophage ratio of 3:1 at 37°C and 5 % CO^2.

Electron Microscopy

To visualize *Leishmania*-infected PMN and the fate of *Leishmania*-infected PMN after uptake by MF, the cells were analysed using structural preservation electron microscopy. For structural preservation electron microscopy, cells were fixed at given time points with 5 % glutaraldehyde for 1 h, treated with 1 % OsO4 for 2 h, and dehydrated in ethanol. The samples were embedded in Araldite (Fluka, Buchs, Switzerland). Ultra-thin sections were contrasted with uranyl acetate and lead citrate and were examined with a Philips EM 400 electron microscope (Eindhoven, The Netherlands).

Generation of Apoptotic PMN

To facilitate neutrophil apoptosis, 350 μl of the freshly isolated neutrophils were irradiated with 256 nm wavelength UV light (200 – 1000 mJ/cm^2) using a Stratalinker (Stratagene, Heidelberg, Germany). Subsequently, irradiated cells were incubated in complete medium for 4 h at 37°C. Double staining with annexin A5 (Roche Molecular Biologicals, Mannheim, Germany) and propidium iodide (PI, Sigma) was used to assess apoptosis and necrosis of the irradiated cells, respectively. Irradiation with 200 mJ/cm^2 UV light led to the generation of cells in early stage of apoptosis, > 80 % of these cells were annexin A5-positive and < 10 % were PI-positive necrotic.

Fluorescent Labelling of Cells

The fluorescent membrane stain PKH67 (green) (Sigma) was used to label freshly isolated neutrophils. 15 x 10^6 cells were washed in serum free RPMI-1640 medium. The pellet was resuspended in 0.5 ml of 5 x 10-7 M PKH67 staining solution and incubated for 5 min at room temperature. After stopping the labelling by adding 0.5 ml of FCS, cells were washed three times with complete medium.

Phagocytosis of apoptotic Neutrophils labelled with a pH sensitive Dye

Apoptotic neutrophils were labelled with the pH sensitive stain pHrodoTM-SE (Invitrogen, Paisley, UK) which emits strong red (532 nm) fluorescence in an acidic (pH 4 - 6) environment and is non-fluorescent at neutral pH. This technique was applied in a recent study to show the engulfment of apoptotic cells by macrophages [58-59]. 25 x 10^6 apoptotic neutrophils in 25 ml PBS were incubated with 20 ng/ml pHrodo-SE at room temperature for 30 min. After washing, labeled apoptotic cells were co-cultured with autologous non-apoptotic neutrophils at a ratio of 4:1 in culture medium containing 30 % autologous serum, 100 ng/ml LPS and 100 U/ml IFN-γ. Cytocentrifuge slides were prepared immediately after mixing the two cell populations or after 90 min of co-culture, mounted and photographed under a fluorescent microscope or with a laser scanning microscope.

REFERENCES

[1]   Pearson RD, Wheeler DA, Harrison LH, Kay HD. The immunobiology of leishmaniasis. Rev Infect Dis 1983; 5:907-27.

[2]   Sharma U, Singh S. Insect vectors of Leishmania: distribution, physiology and their control. J Vector Borne Dis 2008; 45(4):255-72.

[3]   Bogdan C, Rollinghoff M. The immune response to Leishmania: mechanisms of parasite control and evasion. Int J Parasitol 1998; 28(1):121-34.

[4]   Ritter U, Frischknecht F, Van Zandbergen G. Are neutrophils important host cells for Leishmania parasites? Trends Parasitol 2009; 25(11):505-10.

[5]   Bogdan C, Donhauser N, Doring R, Rollinghoff M, Diefenbach A, Rittig MG. Fibroblasts as host cells in latent leishmaniosis. J Exp Med 2000; 191(12):2121-30.

[6]   Laskay T, Van Zandbergen G, Solbach W. Neutrophil granulocytes as host cells and transport vehicles for intracellular pathogens: apoptosis as infection-promoting factor. Immunobiology 2008; 213(3-4):183-91.

[7]   Laufs H, Muller K, Fleischer J, *et al.* Intracellular survival of Leishmania major in neutrophil granulocytes after uptake in the absence of heat-labile serum factors. Infect Immun 2002; 70(2):826-35.

[8]   Nathan C. Neutrophils and immunity: challenges and opportunities. Nat Rev Immunol 2006 Mar;6(3):173-82.

[9]   Scapini P, Lapinet-Vera JA, Gasperini S, Calzetti F, Bazzoni F, Cassatella MA. The neutrophil as a cellular source of chemokines. Immunol Rev 2000; 177:195-203.

[10]   Charmoy M, Brunner-Agten S, Aebischer D, *et al.* Neutrophil-derived CCL3 is essential for the rapid recruitment of dendritic cells to the site of Leishmania major inoculation in resistant mice. PLoS Pathog 2010; 6(2):e1000755.

[11]   Laskay T, Van Zandbergen G, Solbach W. Neutrophil granulocytes--Trojan horses for Leishmania major and other intracellular microbes? Trends Microbiol 2003; 11(5):210-4.

[12]   Peters NC, Egen JG, Secundino N, *et al. In vivo* imaging reveals an essential role for neutrophils in leishmaniasis transmitted by sand flies. Science 2008; 321(5891):970-4.

[13]   Monteiro MC, Nogueira LG, Almeida Souza AA, Ribeiro JM, Silva JS, Cunha FQ. Effect of salivary gland extract of Leishmania vector, Lutzomyia longipalpis, on leukocyte migration in OVA-induced immune peritonitis. Eur J Immunol 2005; 35(8):2424-33.

[14]   Van Zandbergen G, Hermann N, Laufs H, Solbach W, Laskay T. Leishmania promastigotes release a granulocyte chemotactic factor and induce interleukin-8 release but inhibit gamma interferon-inducible protein 10 production by neutrophil granulocytes. Infect Immun 2002; 70(8):4177-84.

[15]   Wenzel A, Van Zandbergen G. Lipoxin A4 receptor dependent leishmania infection. Autoimmunity 2009; 42(4):331-3.

[16]   Ribeiro JM. Role of saliva in blood-feeding by arthropods. Annu Rev Entomol 1987; 32:463-78.:463-78.

[17]   Teixeira CR, Teixeira MJ, Gomes RB, *et al.* Saliva from Lutzomyia longipalpis induces CC chemokine ligand 2/monocyte chemoattractant protein-1 expression and macrophage recruitment. J Immunol 2005; 175(12):8346-53.

[18]   Cougoule C, Constant P, Etienne G, Daffe M, Maridonneau-Parini I. Lack of fusion of azurophil granules with phagosomes during phagocytosis of Mycobacterium smegmatis by human neutrophils is not actively controlled by the bacterium. Infect Immun 2002; 70(3):1591-8.

[19]   Brinkmann V, Reichard U, Goosmann C, *et al.* Neutrophil extracellular traps kill bacteria. Science 2004; 303(5663):1532-5.

[20]   Guimaraes-Costa AB, Nascimento MT, Froment GS, *et al.* Leishmania amazonensis promastigotes induce and are killed by neutrophil extracellular traps. Proc Natl Acad Sci USA 2009; 106(16):6748-53.

[21]   Segal AW. How neutrophils kill microbes. Annu Rev Immunol 2005; 23:197-223.:197-223.

[22]   Fonseca SG, Romao PR, Figueiredo F, *et al.* TNF-alpha mediates the induction of nitric oxide synthase in macrophages but not in neutrophils in experimental cutaneous leishmaniasis. Eur J Immunol 2003; 33(8):2297-306.

[23]   Charmoy M, Megnekou R, Allenbach C, *et al.* Leishmania major induces distinct neutrophil phenotypes in mice that are resistant or susceptible to infection. J Leukoc Biol 2007; 82(2):288-99.

[24]   Perskvist N, Roberg K, Kulyte A, Stendahl O. Rab5a GTPase regulates fusion between pathogen-containing phagosomes and cytoplasmic organelles in human neutrophils. J Cell Sci 2002; 115(Pt 6):1321-30.

[25]   Chen L, Zhang ZH, Watanabe T, *et al.* The involvement of neutrophils in the resistance to Leishmania major infection in susceptible but not in resistant mice. Parasitol Int 2005; 54(2):109-18.

[26]   Ribeiro-Gomes FL, Otero AC, Gomes NA, *et al.* Macrophage interactions with neutrophils regulate Leishmania major infection. J Immunol 2004; 172(7):4454-62.

[27]   Ribeiro-Gomes FL, Moniz-de-Souza MC, Alexandre-Moreira MS, *et al.* Neutrophils activate macrophages for intracellular killing of Leishmania major through recruitment of TLR4 by neutrophil elastase. J Immunol 2007; 179(6):3988-94.

[28]   Gueirard P, Laplante A, Rondeau C, Milon G, Desjardins M. Trafficking of Leishmania donovani promastigotes in non-lytic compartments in neutrophils enables the subsequent transfer of parasites to macrophages. Cell Microbiol 2008; 10(1):100-11.

[29]   Serhan CN, Chiang N, Van Dyke TE. Resolving inflammation: dual anti-inflammatory and pro-resolution lipid mediators. Nat Rev Immunol 2008; 8(5):349-61.

[30]   Godson C, Mitchell S, Harvey K, Petasis NA, Hogg N, Brady HR. Cutting edge: lipoxins rapidly stimulate nonphlogistic phagocytosis of apoptotic neutrophils by monocyte-derived macrophages. J Immunol 2000; 164(4):1663-7.

[31]   Voll RE, Herrmann M, Roth EA, Stach C, Kalden JR, Girkontaite I. Immunosuppressive effects of apoptotic cells. Nature 1997; 390(6658):350-1.

[32]   Meagher LC, Savill JS, Baker A, Fuller RW, Haslett C. Phagocytosis of apoptotic neutrophils does not induce macrophage release of thromboxane B2. J Leukoc Biol 1992; 52(3):269-73.

[33]   Savill JS, Wyllie AH, Henson JE, Walport MJ, Henson PM, Haslett C. Macrophage phagocytosis of aging neutrophils in inflammation. Programmed cell death in the neutrophil leads to its recognition by macrophages. J Clin Invest 1989; 83(3):865-75.

[34]   Van Zandbergen G, Bollinger A, Wenzel A, *et al.* Leishmania disease development depends on the presence of apoptotic promastigotes in the virulent inoculum. Proc Natl Acad Sci U S A 2006; 103(37):13837-42.

[35]   Wanderley JL, Pinto da Silva LH, Deolindo P, *et al.* Cooperation between apoptotic and viable metacyclics enhances the pathogenesis of Leishmaniasis. PLoS One 2009; 4(5):e5733.

[36]   Aga E, Katschinski DM, Van Zandbergen G, *et al.* Inhibition of the spontaneous apoptosis of neutrophil granulocytes by the intracellular parasite Leishmania major. J Immunol 2002; 169(2):898-905.

[37]   Muller K, Van Zandbergen G, Hansen B, *et al.* Chemokines, natural killer cells and granulocytes in the early course of Leishmania major infection in mice. Med Microbiol Immunol 2001; 190(1-2):73-6.

[38]   Allenbach C, Launois P, Mueller C, Tacchini-Cottier F. An essential role for transmembrane TNF in the resolution of the inflammatory lesion induced by Leishmania major infection. Eur J Immunol 2008; 38(3):720-31.

[39]   Erwig LP, Henson PM. Immunological consequences of apoptotic cell phagocytosis. Am J Pathol 2007; 171(1):2-8.

[40]   Fadok VA, Bratton DL, Konowal A, Freed PW, Westcott JY, Henson PM. Macrophages that have ingested apoptotic cells *in vitro* inhibit proinflammatory cytokine production through autocrine/paracrine mechanisms involving TGF-beta, PGE2, and PAF. J Clin Invest 1998; 101(4):890-8.

[41]   Kim S, Elkon KB, Ma X. Transcriptional suppression of interleukin-12 gene expression following phagocytosis of apoptotic cells. Immunity 2004; 21(5):643-53.

[42]   Freire-de-Lima CG, Xiao YQ, Gardai SJ, Bratton DL, Schiemann WP, Henson PM. Apoptotic cells, through transforming growth factor-beta, coordinately induce anti-inflammatory and suppress pro-inflammatory eicosanoid and NO synthesis in murine macrophages. J Biol Chem 2006; 281(50):38376-84.

[43]   Huynh ML, Fadok VA, Henson PM. Phosphatidylserine-dependent ingestion of apoptotic cells promotes TGF-beta1 secretion and the resolution of inflammation. J Clin Invest 2002; 109(1):41-50.

[44]   Esmann L, Idel C, Sarkar A, *et al.* Phagocytosis of apoptotic cells by neutrophil granulocytes: diminished proinflammatory neutrophil functions in the presence of apoptotic cells. J Immunol 2010; 184(1):391-400.

[45]   Dumler JS, Choi KS, Garcia-Garcia JC, *et al.* Human granulocytic anaplasmosis and Anaplasma phagocytophilum. Emerg Infect Dis 2005; 11(12):1828-34.

[46]   Webster P, IJdo JW, Chicoine LM, Fikrig E. The agent of Human Granulocytic Ehrlichiosis resides in an endosomal compartment. J Clin Invest 1998; 101(9):1932-41.

[47]   Rikihisa Y. The tribe Ehrlichieae and ehrlichial diseases. Clin Microbiol Rev 1991; 4(3):286-308.

[48]   Chen SM, Dumler JS, Bakken JS, Walker DH. Identification of a granulocytotropic Ehrlichia species as the etiologic agent of human disease. J Clin Microbiol 1994; 32(3):589-95.

[49]   Mott J, Rikihisa Y. Human granulocytic ehrlichiosis agent inhibits superoxide anion generation by human neutrophils. Infect Immun 2000; 68(12):6697-703.

[50]   Banerjee R, Anguita J, Roos D, Fikrig E. Cutting edge: infection by the agent of human granulocytic ehrlichiosis prevents the respiratory burst by down-regulating gp91phox. J Immunol 2000; 164(8):3946-9.

[51]   IJdo JW, Mueller AC. Neutrophil NADPH oxidase is reduced at the Anaplasma phagocytophilum phagosome. Infect Immun 2004; 72(9):5392-401.

[52]   Carlyon JA, Fikrig E. Mechanisms of evasion of neutrophil killing by Anaplasma phagocytophilum. Curr Opin Hematol 2006; 13(1):28-33.

[53]   Bussmeyer U, Sarkar A, Broszat K, *et al.* Impairment of gamma interferon signaling in human neutrophils infected with Anaplasma phagocytophilum. Infect Immun 2010; 78(1):358-63.

[54]   Ellis TN, Beaman BL. Interferon-gamma activation of polymorphonuclear neutrophil function. Immunology 2004; 112(1):2-12.

[55]   Ray M, Gam AA, Boykins RA, Kenney RT. Inhibition of interferon-gamma signaling by Leishmania donovani. J Infect Dis 2000; 181(3):1121-8.

[56]   Singhal A, Jaiswal A, Arora VK, Prasad HK. Modulation of gamma interferon receptor 1 by Mycobacterium tuberculosis: a potential immune response evasive mechanism. Infect Immun 2007; 75(5):2500-10.

[57]   Vazquez N, Greenwell-Wild T, Rekka S, Orenstein JM, Wahl SM. Mycobacterium avium-induced SOCS contributes to resistance to IFN-gamma-mediated mycobactericidal activity in human macrophages. J Leukoc Biol 2006; 80(5):1136-44.

[58]   Van Zandbergen G, Klinger M, Mueller A, *et al.* Cutting edge: neutrophil granulocyte serves as a vector for Leishmania entry into macrophages. J Immunol 2004; 173(11):6521-5.

[59]   Miksa M, Komura H, Wu R, Shah KG, Wang P. A novel method to determine the engulfment of apoptotic cells by macrophages using pHrodo succinimidyl ester. J Immunol Methods 2009; 342(1-2):71-7.

Index

A

B

C

D

E

F

I

J

L

www.ingramcontent.com/pod-product-compliance
Lightning Source LLC
Chambersburg PA
CBHW050519240326
41598CB00086B/751